D1449552

Recent Advances in Immunization

2nd Edition

Jon Kim Andrus, MD
and
Ciro A. de Quadros, MD, MPH

Editors

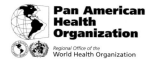

Pan American Health Organization

Regional Office of the
World Health Organization

Pan American Health Organization
Pan American Sanitary Bureau, Regional Office of the
WORLD HEALTH ORGANIZATION
525 Twenty-third Street, N.W.
Washington, D.C. 20037

PAHO HQ Library Cataloguing-in-Publication

Andrus, Jon Kim — ed
    Recent advances in immunization.
Washington, D.C: PAHO, © 2006.
2nd ed.

ISBN 92 7511619 9

I. Title   II. Quadros, Ciro A. de — ed

1. IMMUNIZATION
2. VACCINES, COMBINED
3. BCG VACCINE
4. VACCINATION — trends
5. MEASLES-MUMPS-RUBELLA VACCINE
6. INFLUENZA, HUMAN
7. PAPILLOMAVIRUS, HUMAN

NLM WA 110

CONTENTS

PREFACE

The countries of the Americas, with support from the Pan American Health Organization (PAHO), have made extraordinary progress in providing children with an umbrella of protection against basic, vaccine-preventable diseases. Sustained high levels of national immunization coverage, the eradication of polio, the interruption of endemic measles virus transmission, and the more recent progress towards rubella and congenital rubella syndrome elimination are hemispheric benchmarks of this progress.

In our Region, immunization has been responsible for almost one-quarter of the reduction in mortality in children under 5 years old between 1990 and 2002, contributing significantly to progress toward the Millennium Development Goals and the target of the World Health Organization's Global Immunization Vision and Strategy. These outcomes have been achieved through dedicated country efforts and decades of innovation. Immunization, already regarded as a "best buy" public health intervention, is now believed to have even more far-reaching economic impact, such as in better education outcomes and more years of productive life.

In this context, this book offers national immunization programs continued technical support for the challenges that countries will confront in the years to come. I am delighted to see that issues surrounding combination vaccines, vaccine safety, influenza control, adolescent and adult immunization, BCG vaccine, interpretation of measles and rubella serology, human papillomavirus vaccine, and the approach to the introduction of new vaccines, are all included in this edition. I hope you find the information in this 2nd edition of *Recent Advances in Immunization* as helpful as the first! I want to personally thank the excellent group of experts who served as authors. I especially want to thank the editors, Drs. Jon Andrus and Ciro de Quadros, for all their initiative, hard work, and commitment in putting this updated PAHO publication together.

Dr. Mirta Roses Periago
Director

INTRODUCTION

The first edition of *Recent Advances in Immunization* was published by the Pan American Health Organization in 1983. Today, twenty-three years later, the editors are pleased to be able to provide this second edition. We believe this reissue comes at a critical time in the evolution of national immunization programs. Immunization is at a crossroads. The future offers new opportunities to tackle important public health priorities with new technologies. However, new vaccines are much more expensive than the traditional vaccines used in childhood immunization programs. Evidence-based, informed decisions will be critical for sustaining the success of immunization.

The first edition was grounded in the principles of the Expanded Program on Immunization (EPI). The September 1978 Declaration of Alma-Ata highlighted EPI as an essential component of primary and maternal-and-child health care. When it was originally launched in the Americas, EPI spearheaded the following long-term objectives:

- reducing morbidity and mortality from diphtheria, tetanus, pertussis, measles, poliomyelitis, and tuberculosis by providing immunization against these diseases to all children by 1990;
- promoting the countries' self-reliance in the delivery of immunization services as a part of their general health services; and
- promoting regional self-reliance in the production and quality control of vaccines.

Thanks to the work of immunization programs throughout the Region's countries, the peoples of the Americas now live free of indigenous polio and measles; neonatal tetanus, diphtheria, and pertussis have been well-controlled; and new vaccines have been added to national immunization programs and their application has been sustained. As a result, high coverage levels have been achieved for the diseases originally covered by EPI, as well as for hepatitis B, rubella, mumps, and *Haemophilus influenzae*. In September 2003, the Directing Council of PAHO launched the regional initiative to eliminate rubella and congenital rubella syndrome in the Americas by the year 2010.

Undeniably, progress has been extraordinary—diseases have been eradicated or eliminated and the public health infrastructure has been strengthened—but progress has been uneven. Some countries still have a significant proportion of their populations living in districts where coverage remains below 95%. Sporadic outbreaks of diphtheria and pertussis still occur because of an accumulation of susceptibles missed by routine national programs. This accumulation of susceptibles also puts countries at risk for large measles outbreaks when importations of measles virus occur, as has recently happened in Mexico (2003–2004), Venezuela (2001–2002), and Colombia (2002).

These remaining challenges point to the need to complete the unfinished agenda. Reaching children and families who live in low-coverage areas will be essential for sustaining the success of measles elimination and for achieving the targets to eliminate rubella and congenital rubella syndrome. Improving surveillance of vaccine preventable diseases also is a key underpinning of this strategy.

This unfinished agenda also must embrace other global initiatives such as the Millennium Development Goals (MDGs) and the targets outlined in World Health Organization's Global Immunization Vision and Strategy (GIVS). To reach the targets, some countries will need to seriously consider the introduction of new or underutilized life-saving vaccines. Vaccines targeting diseases caused by pneumococcus, rotavirus, human papilloma virus, and influenza may greatly help in reaching the MDGs and GIVS. Reaching these targets also will require that immunization programs evolve from targeting just children to including the whole family. Including the whole family will enable countries to attain higher vaccination coverage of adolescents and adults for influenza and human papilloma virus, as well as for human immunodeficiency virus and other diseases when future vaccines against them become available.

Some countries will have to overcome extraordinary technical and programmatic challenges if they are to complete this unfinished agenda. The chapters in this 2nd edition attempt to address some of them. Before embarking on the design and preparation of this book, we surveyed the countries of the Americas to compile a list of the most relevant topics that countries face in trying to deliver high-quality immunization services. The information collected provided the framework for the topics addressed by the chapters in this book. To that end, this book is intended to primarliy assist national immunization managers and their staff with their program of work. However, we expect many other health professionals and other groups to benefit, including students of schools of public health, medicine, and nursing; epidemiologists and disease control specialists; experts on surveillance of vaccine preventable diseases; vaccinologists; and infectologists. The first edition was translated into multiple languages and was distributed worldwide. We hope this edition can provide the same degree of support to national immunization programs and any other interested user.

The list of authors and co-authors participating in the writing of this book is impressive. We are honored to have worked with this distinguished group of colleagues who bring with them the necessary scientific expertise, as well as the critical field experience.

Jon Kim Andrus, M.D.
Lead Technical Advisor, Immunization Unit
Pan American Health Organization

and

Ciro A. de Quadros, M.D., M.P.H.
Director of International Programs
Albert B. Sabin Vaccine Institute

Editors

ACKNOWLEDGMENTS

The authors would like to dedicate this book to all the national immunization program managers and their staff, who so tirelessly work on behalf of the world's children and their families. To have had the chance to work with them over the years around the world has been an honor.

We also want to recognize several people for their support in preparing this book. Dr. Neal A. Halsey reviewed the chapter on combination vaccines and participated in the initial discussions on the book's format. Dr. Rachel Rodin helped with vaccine literature searches. Ms. Cecilia Parker edited the publication. Ms. Nisha Aravindakshan and Ms. Diana Picón oversaw production and layout of this book.

ADOLESCENT AND ADULT IMMUNIZATION

Cristiana M. Toscano, MD, PhD,[1] *Jarbas Barbosa da Silva Jr., MD, MPH, PhD,*[2] *and Stanley Plotkin, MD*[3]

INTRODUCTION

Immunization strategies and policies worldwide have primarily targeted children, and the effective implementation of childhood vaccination programs has resulted in the substantial decline in the occurrence of many vaccine-preventable diseases in almost all countries and regions of the world.

This success notwithstanding, childhood vaccination clearly has not been able to completely control vaccine-preventable diseases, because a significant proportion of morbidity and mortality occurs among adolescents and adults. Persons who were not naturally infected or who were not vaccinated are at risk, constituting a susceptible group in which circulation of some of these agents may continue indefinitely, even when high vaccination coverages in children are achieved.

In addition, certain epidemiologic characteristics such as age, occupation, environment, lifestyle, and special health problems are important risk factors for certain vaccine-preventable diseases. Vaccination recommendations should consider these as well as other variables, such as the individual's susceptibility, risk of exposure to the disease, complications of the disease, and benefits and risks of the immunizing agent.

[1] EPI Consultant, Immunization Unit, Pan American Health Organization.
[2] Ministry of Health, Brazil.
[3] University of Pennsylvania, Wistar Institute, Sanofi Pasteur.

MAIN FACTORS INFLUENCING VACCINATION IN ADULTS AND ADOLESCENTS

In general there is little knowledge or awareness about the burden of vaccine-preventable disease in adult populations and in populations at risk. Moreover, new life-saving vaccines are costly, which makes it difficult to prioritize their introduction if there are budget constraints. Even when the vaccines are available and recommended, operational difficulties in vaccinating adolescents, adults, and specific high-risk groups frequently result in low coverage levels. Mobilizing older populations is difficult, and few countries, with the exception of countries in the Americas in terms of rubella elimination strategies, have the experience of mass vaccination of adults. Health care providers' missed opportunities to vaccinate adults during office, clinic, or hospital visits also must be addressed. This chapter seeks to provide evidence for decision making with regard to controversial aspects of adult and adolescent immunization.

Specific vaccines that should be considered for adults as primary or booster vaccines include vaccines against measles/mumps/rubella, influenza, pneumococcal infections, diphtheria/tetanus toxoids, and hepatitis B. Yellow fever vaccination should be part of vaccination series in areas of risk. New vaccines for inclusion in adolescent and adult schedules include meningococcal, pertussis, and human papillomavirus vaccines. In the future, vaccines against sexually transmitted diseases and against congenital infections also may be considered.

INFLUENZA VACCINATION IN ADULTS

Influenza is covered in detail in another chapter; this section will only highlight key aspects of adult vaccination. Influenza viruses are responsible for major epidemics of respiratory disease worldwide, which are associated with high incidence of acute illness and respiratory complications resulting in high morbidity and mortality. The risks for complications, hospitalization, and death from influenza have been demonstrated to be higher among persons aged ≥65 years, young children, and persons with certain underlying health conditions regardless of age (1). Estimated rates of influenza-associated hospitalizations vary substantially by age group, being higher at extremes of age (<1 and ≥65 years old) (2, 3). Influenza-related mortality can result from pneumonia and from cardiopulmonary disease. Older adults account for ≥90% of deaths attributed to pneumonia and influenza (4, 5).

The use of influenza vaccine is the most important measure in preventing influenza infection and its complications. Both inactivated influenza vaccine and live, attenuated influenza vaccine are available for use. The most widely used influenza vaccine is the fractioned inactivated vaccine. The live vaccine has been licensed for use in the United States in children and healthy adults aged 5–49 years since 2003, and it is administered intranasally. Its safety for other age groups is under evaluation.

Currently used influenza vaccines contain three virus strains identified by a global surveillance network as the strains circulating worldwide. They are composed of influenza A subtypes H1N1 and H3N2, and influenza type B. Two recommendations for the vaccine composition are made annually by the World Health Organization: one each for the southern and northern hemispheres.

The effectiveness of inactivated influenza vaccine depends primarily on age, underlying immunologic conditions, and similarity between the circulating viruses and those present in the vaccine. Nearly all vaccinated young adults develop high post-vaccination antibody titers (6, 7). When the vaccine and circulating viruses are antigenically similar, the influenza vaccine prevents influenza illness among approximately 70%–90% of healthy adults aged <65 years (8–10). Vaccination of healthy adults has resulted in decreased work absenteeism when the vaccine and circulating viruses are well-matched (8–11).

Lower post-vaccination antibody titers are developed in older persons and in those with certain chronic diseases (12–13). Vaccine efficacy of 58% against influenza respiratory illness has been demonstrated in non-institutionalized persons aged ≥60 years, but efficacy might be lower among those aged ≥70 years (14). Other studies have demonstrated 30%–70% effectiveness in preventing hospitalization for pneumonia and influenza among non-institutionalized elderly (15, 16).

Vaccination against influenza in elderly persons ≥ 65 years of age is effective in preventing secondary complications and reducing the risk of influenza-related hospitalization and death (16–19). A recent study demonstrated that vaccination in the elderly was associated with a reduction of 19% in the risk of hospitalization for cardiac disease, 16%–23% for cerebrovascular disease, and 29%–32% for pneumonia or influenza. In addition, a 48%–50% reduction in the risk of death from all causes was demonstrated (20). These data strongly support efforts to increase the rates of vaccination among the elderly.

Among older persons who reside in nursing homes, influenza vaccine is most effective in preventing severe illness, secondary complications, and deaths. In this population, the vaccine can be 50%–60% effective in preventing hospitalization or pneumonia and 80% effective in preventing death, although the effectiveness in preventing influenza illness often ranges from 30% to 40% (17–21).

Cost-effectiveness Studies of Influenza Vaccination

Studies on the cost-effectiveness of influenza vaccination can provide important information to guide decision making. Most studies demonstrate that influenza vaccination reduces health-care costs and productivity losses associated with influenza illness. Economic studies of influenza vaccination of persons aged >65 years conducted in the United States have reported overall cost savings and substantial reductions in hospitalization and death (15, 16, 22). Studies of adults aged <65 years have reported that vaccination can reduce both direct medical costs and indirect costs from work absenteeism (9, 10, 23–25).

Cost-effectiveness results depend on the influenza attack rate, vaccine effectiveness, and vaccination cost. One cost-effectiveness analysis estimated a cost ranging from $60–$4,000/illness averted among healthy persons aged 18–64 years (10). A cost-benefit economic model estimated an average annual savings of $13.66/person vaccinated (26). In this study, 78% of all costs prevented were costs from lost work productivity, whereas the first study did not include productivity losses from influenza illness. These different results indicate that it is important to consider the methods used in different studies when analyzing their results.

Economic studies specifically evaluating the cost-effectiveness of vaccinating persons aged 50–64 years old are not available, and the number of studies that examine the economics of routinely vaccinating children with inactivated or live, attenuated vaccine are limited. However, in a study of inactivated vaccine that included all age groups, cost utility improved with increasing age and among those with chronic medical conditions, with vaccination resulting in net savings per quality-adjusted life years (QALYs) gained among persons aged >65 years (27).

Additional studies of the relative cost-effectiveness and cost utility of influenza vaccination among children and among adults aged <65 years are needed and should be designed to account for year-to-year variations in influenza attack rates, illness severity, and vaccine efficacy when evaluating the long-term costs and benefits of annual vaccination.

Duration of Immunity and Vaccine Schedule

Influenza vaccine should be administered annually, before the influenza season. This recommendation is based both in the fact that circulating strains change annually in each epidemic period, as well as evidence that immunity declines during the year after vaccination (28, 29). Therefore, even when the current influenza vaccine contains one or more antigens administered in previous years, annual vaccination with the current vaccine is necessary. When planning for vaccination campaigns, it should be taken into consideration that adults develop peak antibody protection against influenza infection two weeks after vaccination (*30, 31*). Vaccine prepared for a previous influenza season should not be administered to provide protection for the current season.

Vaccination Indications

Considering the evidence presented above regarding morbidity and mortality associated with influenza, vaccine effectiveness, and economic analysis, these are the groups of adolescents and adults which would benefit most from vaccination, due to increased risk for influenza infection and complications:

- all individuals aged ≥65 years and
- adults and children with clinical conditions predisposing them to higher risk of lower-respiratory-tract complications and death after influenza infection. These individuals have been identified as those with chronic disorders of the cardiovascular, pulmonary, and/or renal systems (including asthma); with metabolic diseases (including diabetes mellitus); with severe anemia; with hemoglobinopathies; and/or with compromised immune function, including HIV infection.

Health-care providers, caregivers, and household members caring for high-risk persons may transmit influenza infections to their high-risk patients while they themselves are incubating an infection, undergoing a subclinical infection, or having mild symptoms. Nosocomial outbreaks of influenza have been reported, and evidence indicates that vaccination of health-care personnel is associated with decreased deaths among nursing home patients (*32, 33*). Since some high-risk persons can have relatively low antibody responses to influenza vaccine, the potential for introducing influenza into a high-risk group should be reduced by targeted vaccination programs of medical personnel. Therefore, the following groups also should be considered for vaccination:

- physicians, nurses, and other personnel in hospitals or outpatient care settings who have contact with high-risk patients in all age groups, including infants;
- employees of nursing homes and chronic-care facilities who have contact with patients or residents;
- providers of home care to high-risk persons; and
- household members (including children) of high-risk persons.

Studies indicate that rates of hospitalization are higher among young children than older children when influenza viruses are in circulation (*2, 3*), and these rates are comparable to those of other groups considered at high risk for influenza-related complications. Because children <2 years are at increased risk for influenza-related hospitalization (2, 3, 34), children aged 6 months to 2 years of age should also be vaccinated. In addition, vaccination is recommended for their household contacts and out-of-home caregivers, particularly for contacts of children aged 0–5 months, because influenza vaccines are not licensed for use among children aged <6 months.

Types of Vaccine

Healthy persons aged 5–49 years in these groups who are not contacts of severely immunosuppressed persons can receive either attenuated or inactivated influenza vaccine. All other persons in this group should receive inactivated influenza vaccine. The rationale for not using attenuated vaccine among health-care workers caring for immunosuppressed patients is the theoretical risk that a live-vaccine virus could be transmitted to severely immunosuppressed persons. Recommendation for live vaccine use may change as additional data are acquired. Either vaccine may be administered to health-care workers or other adults who care for, or have close contact with, immunosuppressed individuals or with other groups at high risk.

Dosage and Route

Dosage recommendations vary according to age group. Among adults, studies have indicated limited or no improvement in antibody response when a second dose is administered during the same season (31, 35, 36). The intramuscular route is recommended for influenza vaccine. Adults should be vaccinated in the deltoid muscle. A needle length ≥1 inch can be used, because needles <1 inch might not be long enough to penetrate muscle tissue in certain adults and older children (37).

Influenza Vaccination in the Americas

Countries in the Americas are progressively introducing vaccination against influenza targeting priority groups (Table 1). Limited data on viral circulation patterns in equatorial regions are available. Further studies are needed to evaluate epidemic periods in these regions and guide decision-makers regarding vaccine use and vaccination periods.

PNEUMOCOCCAL VACCINATION IN ADULTS

Currently available pneumococcal vaccines are the polysaccharide 23-valent vaccine and conjugate vaccines (7, 9, 11-valent). The polysaccharide

TABLE 1. Countries offering influenza vaccine in the public sector, by year of vaccine introduction and target population, Region of the Americas, 2004–2005.

Country	Year of introduction	Target population	2004 coverage (%)	2005 coverage (%)
Bermuda	1970s	Over 6 months to 18 years	...	...
		Over 50 years	...	...
		Over 65 years	59	64
		Persons with chronic diseases	...	...
		Health workers	...	...
		Pregnant women (>10 weeks)	...	...
Chile	1975	Over 65 years	97	95
		Persons with chronic diseases	100	100
		Pregnant women	58	94
		Health workers	100	100
		Over 6 months to 5 years with chronic disease	...	...
Cayman Islands	1990	Over 6 months to 5 years	...	...
		Over 50 years	...	...
		Persons with chronic diseases	...	...
		Health workers	...	...
		Pregnant women[a]	...	...
Argentina	1993	Over 65 years	...	...
		Persons with chronic diseases	...	...
		Health workers	...	...
Cuba	1998	Over 60 years in homes	100	100
		Over 85 years old	...	100
		Persons with chronic disease	100	100
		Health workers in National Reference Laboratory	100	100
		Persons who work with birds	100	100
		Persons with HIV	100	100
		Persons with physical/mental disability	100	100
		Other groups	100	100
Uruguay	1998	Over 6 months to 2 years	15	<15
		Over 24 months with risk factors	...	...
		Older adults	...	...
		Persons with chronic diseases	...	...
		Health workers	...	...
		Pregnant women	...	...
Brazil	1999	Over 60 years	91	88
		Persons with chronic diseases	...	...
		Health workers	...	...
		Other risk groups (including indigenous and incarcerated)	...	...

(Table continues on next page)

TABLE 1. (Continued).

Country	Year of introduction	Target population	2004 coverage (%)	2005 coverage (%)
Netherland Antilles (Saba)	1999	Persons over 65 years	...	...
		Persons with chronic disease	...	...
		Health workers	...	...
		Pregnant women	...	...
British Virgin Islands	2000	Elderly home residents	33	0
		Persons with renal dysfunction	90	90
Honduras	2003	Children 6 months to 23 months with chronic disease	...	...
		Persons over 60 years	100	100
		Health workers	100	100
		Persons working in poultry farms	...	100
Costa Rica	2004	6 months to 5 years with chronic diseases	88	...
		Over 65 years	98	...
El Salvador	2004	6 months to 23 months	70[b]	77[c]
		Persons over 60 years	99[b]	96[c]
		Persons with chronic diseases	...	...
		Health workers	85[b]	...
Mexico	2004	Over 6 months to 23 months	...	...
		Over 60 years	...	70
		Over 65 years	...	85
		Persons with chronic diseases	...	...
		Health workers	...	...
Anguilla	2005	Elderly with chronic diseases	...	51
		Health workers	...	51
Bahamas	2005	Over 6 months to 5 years	...	...
		Over 65 years	...	...
		Persons with chronic diseases	...	...
		Health workers	...	...
Colombia	2005	Children 6 months to 23 months	...	...
		Children 6 months to 18 months with respiratory disease or living in poor areas	...	10
		Over 65 years old	...	...
		Over 65 and institutionalized	...	10
Panama	2005	Children 7 months to 23 months	...	...
		Persons over 60 years	...	100
		Persons with chronic disease	...	...
		Health workers	...	...

TABLE 1. (Continued).

Country	Year of introduction	Target population	2004 coverage (%)	2005 coverage (%)
Paraguay	2005	Persons over 60 years	...	13
		Persons with pulmonary disease	...	23
		Persons with cardiovascular disease	...	8
		Persons with diabetes	...	32
		Persons with renal dysfunction	...	34
		Persons with immunosuppressive disease	...	6
		Health workers	...	36
		Bird breeders and persons providing essential services	...	12
French Guiana	...	Over 65 years	...	...
		Persons with chronic disease	...	...
		Health workers	...	...

[a] On doctor's recommendation.
[b] Coverage assessed in January 2005.
[c] Coverage assessed in December 2005.
... Data not available.

Sources: Country Survey, 2006; Canada and the United States are not included. Ropero AM, Oliva O, Picón D, Gilani Z, Andrus JK. Update on the status of influenza vaccination in the Region of the Americas. Abstract presented at the XVII Technical Advisory Group (TAG) Meeting on Vaccine-preventable Diseases. Pan American Health Organization. July 25th–27th, Guatemala City, Guatemala, 2006.

vaccine is composed of 23 purified capsular polysaccharide antigens of *S. pneumoniae* (serotypes 1, 2, 3, 4, 5, 6B, 7F, 8, 9N, 9V, 10A, 11A, 12F, 14, 15B, 17F, 18C, 19A, 19F, 20, 22F, 23F, and 33F). This vaccine was developed in the 1980s and replaced an earlier 14-valent formulation. The 23 capsular types in the vaccine represent at least 85%–90% of the serotypes that cause invasive pneumococcal infections among children and adults in the United States. The six serotypes (6B, 9V, 14, 19A, 19F, and 23F) that most frequently cause invasive drug-resistant pneumococcal infection in the United States are represented in the 23-valent vaccine (*38*).

The development of a protein-polysaccharide conjugate vaccine for selected serotypes is aimed at improved immunogenicity and protective efficacy of pneumococcal vaccination, particularly in children under 2 years old. In this age group, incidence of disease is higher and antibody responses to the polysaccharide vaccine are poor (*38*). Conjugation of polysaccharides to proteins changes the anti-polysaccharide immune response from B cells only to T and B cells, leading to a substantial primary response among infants and a strong booster response at re-exposure (*39*).

In 2000, the 7-valent pneumococcal conjugate vaccine was licensed in several countries worldwide. The 7-valent conjugate vaccine contains serotypes 4, 6B, 9V, 14, 18C, 19F, and 23F. In addition to providing protection to children aged <2 years, conjugate vaccine decreases nasopharyngeal colonization, a substantial source of transmission of pneumococci (40–41).

Disease Burden

The highest rates of invasive pneumococcal disease occur among young children, especially those aged <2 years (38). Incidence among persons of all ages and among persons aged ≥65 years was 24 per 100,000 and 61 per 100,000 in 1998, respectively (42).

Pneumococcal infections are associated with high mortality worldwide. Case-fatality rates are highest for meningitis and bacteremia. The highest age-specific mortality occurs among the elderly. Despite appropriate antimicrobial therapy and intensive medical care, the overall case-fatality rate for pneumococcal bacteremia is 15%–20% among adults, and approximately 30%–40% among elderly patients (43–45). An overall case-fatality rate of 36% was documented for adult, inner-city residents who were hospitalized for pneumococcal bacteremia (46).

Persons who have certain underlying medical conditions are at increased risk for developing pneumococcal infection or experiencing severe disease and complications. Adults at increased risk include those who are generally immunocompetent but who have chronic cardiovascular diseases (e.g., congestive heart failure or cardiomyopathy), chronic pulmonary diseases (e.g., chronic obstructive pulmonary disease or emphysema), or chronic liver diseases (e.g., cirrhosis). Diabetes mellitus often is associated with cardiovascular or renal dysfunction, which increases the risk for severe pneumococcal illness. The incidence of pneumococcal infection is increased for persons who have liver disease as a result of alcohol abuse (38). Asthma has not been associated with an increased risk for pneumococcal disease, unless it occurs with chronic bronchitis, emphysema, or long-term use of systemic corticosteroids. Functional or anatomic asplenia (e.g., sickle cell disease or splenectomy) is also associated with higher risk for pneumococcal infection.

In addition, immunosuppressive conditions leading to a decreased responsiveness to polysaccharide antigens or increased rate of decline in serum antibody concentrations are risk factors for developing pneumococcal infection. These include conditions such as congenital immunodeficiency, human immunodeficiency virus infection, leukemia, lymphoma, multiple myeloma, Hodgkin's disease, or generalized malignancy; organ or bone marrow transplantation; therapy with alkylating agents, antimetabolites, or systemic corticosteroids; or chronic renal failure or nephrotic syndrome. As many as 91% of adults who have invasive pneumococcal infection have at least one of the previously mentioned underlying medical conditions, or are of an age greater than or equal to 65 years (44, 47, 48).

Duration of Antibody Levels

Levels of antibodies to most pneumococcal vaccine antigens remain elevated for at least five years in healthy adults. In some, antibody concentrations decrease to prevaccination levels by 10 years (49). A more rapid decline (i.e., within 5–10 years after vaccination) in antibody concentrations may occur in elderly persons, persons who have undergone splenectomy, patients with renal disease requiring dialysis, patients with Hodgkin's disease and multiple myeloma, and persons who have received transplants (49–54). However, quantitative measurements of antibodies do not account for the quality of the antibody being produced, and functional immune response may ultimately be more relevant for evaluating response to pneumococcal vaccination (38).

Vaccine Efficacy

Several clinical trials have been conducted evaluating the efficacy of vaccine against pneumonia and pneumococcal bacteremia, and some case-control and serotype prevalence studies have provided evidence for effectiveness against invasive disease. Various studies, including one meta-analysis of nine randomized controlled trials, have demonstrated an absent protective effect of the polysaccharide pneumococcal vaccine for nonbacteremic pneumonia among persons in high-risk groups (38, 55). This same meta-analysis concluded that pneumococcal vaccine is efficacious in reducing the frequency of bacteremic pneumococcal pneumonia among adults in low-risk groups (55). However, the vaccine is not effective in preventing disease caused by non-vaccine serotype organisms (56).

Effectiveness against invasive diseases in case-control studies ranges from 56% to 81% (38). Vaccine effectiveness of 65%–84% also was demonstrated among specific high-risk groups. Effectiveness in immunocompetent individuals 65 years of age or older was 75%.

A recent retrospective cohort study involving more than 47,000 persons aged 65 years or older evaluated the effectiveness of pneumococcal polysaccharide vaccine against community-acquired pneumonia, as well as the more specific outcome of pneumococcal bacteremia (57). Results indicated that vaccination was associated with a 44% reduction in the risk of pneumococcal bacteremia, but there was no association between vaccination and all cases of community-acquired pneumonia.

Considering the known impact of conjugate vaccine in decreasing nasopharyngeal colonization as a source of transmission of pneumococci in the community, a recent study was conducted to evaluate whether the incidence of invasive pneumococcal disease among adults aged 50 years or older had changed in the four years since pneumococcal conjugate vaccine was introduced in the United States (*58*). Incidence of invasive pneumococcal disease among adults aged 50 years or older declined 28% (40.8 cases per 100,000 in 1998–1999 to 29.4 in 2002–2003), resulting from indirect vaccine effects benefiting older adults.

Cost-effectiveness Studies

Several studies have evaluated the cost-effectiveness of pneumococcal polysaccharide vaccine in the elderly population. Some studies suggest that routine vaccination of all elderly persons with the 23-valent pneumococcal polysaccharide vaccine is more cost-effective than the strategy adopted by several countries of vaccinating high-risk groups (*59, 60*). When comparing influenza and pneumococcal vaccination for those aged 65 and older, costs for the prevention of one hospitalization or death each year were similar in both programs (*60*).

Different cost-effectiveness studies evaluating vaccination of the elderly have shown results varying from cost-savings (negative values of US$ per life-year gained) to 33,000 Euros per life-year gained, when compared to other health-care strategies currently in place (*61*). Results varied according to vaccine efficacy estimates, being more cost-effective when higher effectiveness among specific populations were considered.

As several guidelines recommend pneumococcal vaccination starting at age 50, one study compared cost-effectiveness of vaccinating black and non-black persons 50–65 years old. Results indicate a much higher cost-effective ratio in the higher risk black population, supporting the current recommendation to vaccinate high-risk people in this age group (*62*). Vaccination of healthy younger adults with pneumococcal vaccine is not a cost-effective strategy (*63*).

Vaccine Indications

The use of pneumococcal polysaccharide vaccine has been recommended by many different countries, and has been consistently recommended by several medical societies worldwide. In light of recent evidence, the following recommendations may be considered when developing policies for pneumococcal vaccination. Vaccinate:

- all individuals aged ≥65 years.
- adults younger than 65 years who are at increased risk for pneumococcal disease or its complications. Persons at increased risk for severe disease include those with chronic illness such as chronic cardiovascu-

lar disease, chronic pulmonary disease, diabetes mellitus, alcoholism, chronic liver disease, or cerebrospinal fluid leaks. In addition, all individuals with functional or anatomic asplenia, or decreased immunologic function should be vaccinated.
• Persons with asymptomatic or symptomatic HIV infection as soon as possible after their diagnosis is confirmed.

The importance of surveillance activities in the Region cannot be overstated, including strengthening overall laboratory capacity, as well as clinical and epidemiological components. In addition to conducting economic analysis evaluation, key surveillance centers should conduct surveillance of pneumococcal disease in adults, thereby strengthening its population-based component as a way to support and document the impact of vaccination.

Revaccination

Data estimating serologic correlates of protection are not conclusive. The overall increase in antibody levels among elderly persons has been determined to be lower after revaccination than following primary vaccination (*64, 65*). However, revaccination after 5–10 years has been demonstrated to be safe and induces significant immune response in most persons (*65*).

Revaccination in chronically ill, older, nursing-facility residents at least five years after primary vaccination was associated with a significant but brief immunological response for most of the serotypes tested (*66*). Long-term follow-up data concerning antibody levels in persons who have been revaccinated are still pending.

Although one study has suggested that vaccination may provide protection for at least nine years after the initial dose (*67*), another study demonstrated decreasing estimates of effectiveness with increasing time, particularly among those older than 85 years (*56*).

Considering this, revaccination is recommended for those who are at highest risk for serious pneumococcal infection and those who are likely to have a rapid decline in pneumococcal antibody levels, provided that five years have elapsed since the first dose of pneumococcal vaccine was administered. Those aged 65 years and older should be given a second vaccine dose if they have not received the vaccine within five years and received the primary vaccination before the age of 65.

The need for subsequent doses of pneumococcal vaccine is unclear and should be assessed as additional data become available. Because data are insufficient concerning the safety of pneumococcal vaccine when administered three or more times, revaccination following a second dose is not routinely recommended.

Research into conjugate- and protein-based pneumococcal vaccines that induce immunologic memory is needed in older persons and among adults at increased risk for pneumococcal infection. Benefits and risks involved with using a 7-, 9-, 11-, or 15-valent pneumococcal conjugate vaccine in place of, or in addition to, polysaccharide 23-valent vaccine have not yet been established.

DIPHTHERIA AND TETANUS VACCINATION IN ADULTS

The occurrence of diphtheria has decreased dramatically in the Americas, largely due to the widespread use of diphtheria toxoid and increased vaccination coverage in the population aged < 1 year (Figure 1). Only about 50 cases of respiratory diphtheria were reported in 2003 in the Region. Recent outbreaks in Ecuador (1993–1994), Colombia (2000), Paraguay (2002), and Haiti (2004) that predominantly affected adolescents and older children were associated with low vaccine coverage rates and incomplete vaccination. These outbreaks were controlled through vaccination of children and susceptible adults at risk (Table 2).

The number of tetanus cases in the Americas also has decreased in past decades. Nevertheless, 881 cases of accidental tetanus were notified in the Region in 2003 and 825 cases were notified in 2004. The vast majority of these cases occurred in persons 15 years or older. Tetanus occurs almost exclusively among unvaccinated or inadequately vaccinated persons. Teta-

FIGURE 1. Number of reported diphtheria and pertussis cases and DPT3 coverage in children <1 year old, Region of the Americas, 1978–2004.

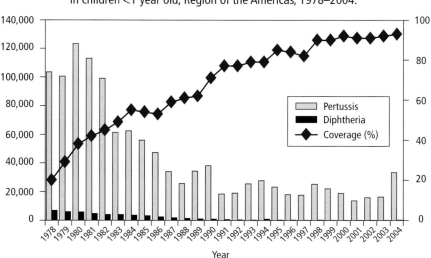

Year

Source: Immunization Unit, Pan American Health Organization.

TABLE 2. Recent diphtheria outbreaks, selected countries in the Americas, 1993–2002.[a, b]

	Countries		
	Ecuador	Colombia	Paraguay
Year	1993 and 1994	2000	2002
Number of cases	724	12	50[c]
Case-fatality rate	No data	12%	15%
Vaccination coverage	Low coverage	Decreased coverage	Low coverage
Performance of the surveillance system	Improved response in the 1994 outbreak	Adequate	Problems in case notification and delay in implementing control measures
Vaccination status of the cases	15% unvaccinated; 22% referred having some prior doses (no documentation); no information for the remaining cases	62% with incomplete vaccination schedule	74% without vaccination history
Most affected age group	86% in individuals aged 15 years and older	50% in individuals aged 5–9 years	57% in individuals aged 5–14 years
Socioeconomic status/living environment	Low; urban slums	Low; urban slums	Low; urban slums
Control measures taken	Vaccination of children younger than 5 years of age; booster dose; vaccination of adults at risk	Vaccination of children younger than 5 years of age; booster dose; vaccination of adults at risk	Vaccination of children younger than 5 years of age; booster dose; vaccination of adults at risk

[a] Data source: country reports, PAHO.
[b] Data from outbreak in Haiti and Dominican Republic (2004) not included in the table.
[c] Cases updated as of week 40, 2002.

Source: Ropero AM, Oliva O, Castillo-Solorzano C, Dietz V, Izurieta H, Carrasco P, et al. Recent outbreaks of diphtheria in the Americas. Abstract presented at the XV Technical Advisory Group (TAG) Meeting on Vaccine-preventable Diseases. Pan American Health Organization. November 22nd–23rd, Washington, D.C., 2002.

nus toxoid is safe, inexpensive, effective, and widely available in most countries. Therefore, special efforts should be directed towards vaccinating unvaccinated or inadequately vaccinated adolescents and adults, particularly pregnant women.

Complete and appropriately timed vaccination is at least 85% effective in preventing diphtheria. The combined tetanus and diphtheria toxoids adsorbed for adult use (Td) is recommended for use among persons

7 years old or older, because a large proportion of them lack protective levels of circulating antibody against tetanus (*68*).

After complete and adequately timed vaccination, tetanus toxoid is nearly 100% effective in preventing tetanus. Td is the preferred preparation for active tetanus immunization of persons greater than or equal to 7 years of age because a large proportion of them also lack protective levels of circulating antitoxin against diphtheria (*69–72*).

All adults lacking a completed primary series of diphtheria and tetanus toxoids should complete the series with Td. A primary series for adults is three doses of preparations containing diphtheria and tetanus toxoids, with the first two doses given at least four weeks apart and the third dose given 6–12 months after the second. All adults for whom 10 years or more have elapsed since completion of their primary series or since their last booster dose should receive a dose of Td. Thereafter, a booster dose of Td should be administered every 10 years. There is no need to repeat doses if the schedule for the primary series or booster doses is delayed.

In many countries the routine diphtheria, tetanus, and pertussis (DPT) pediatric vaccination schedule (children <7 years of age) includes four doses at 2, 4, 6, and 15 months of age, and a booster dose at age 4–6 years, before entering kindergarten or elementary school. The first Td booster should be done at age 14–16 years (10 years after the dose administered at age 4–6 years).

MEASLES, MUMPS, AND RUBELLA VACCINATION IN ADULTS

The Region of the Americas is targeting measles eradication, and only imported cases have been identified in the Region since 2002 (Figure 2). Every country, except Haiti, has introduced the combined measles, mumps, and rubella (MMR) vaccine into its immunization program for children 9–12 months of age. In areas with endemic measles circulation, adolescents and adults not vaccinated have already been exposed to the disease and therefore are immune. Considering the risk of importation of measles cases from endemic regions of the world, specific groups with higher risk of exposure to imported cases should be targeted for vaccination, including travelers, health care workers, tourism industry workers, and sex workers.

Measles and Mumps

Although children in many developing countries will have high rates of natural immunity to these infections, wherever measles elimination is the goal, mass vaccination is often undertaken. If financially possible, the vaccine used should be the MMR combination, in order to achieve maximum public health effect.

FIGURE 2. Measles cases and vaccine coverage of 1-year-old children, Region of the Americas, 1990–2004.

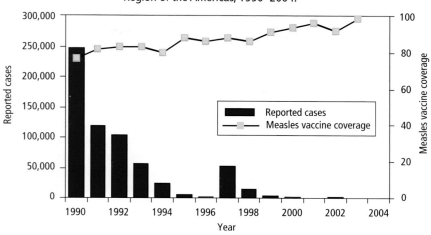

Source: Immunization Unit, Pan American Health Organization.

Rubella

About half of the world's countries use rubella vaccine, almost always in combination with measles or measles and mumps vaccines (*73*). Routine vaccination of children will ultimately prevent rubella in adults through herd immunity and the eventual aging of the vaccinated cohort into adulthood, as demonstrated by rubella elimination efforts in North America (*74*) and the Scandinavian countries (*75, 76*).

In September 2003, the countries of the Americas adopted a resolution to eliminate rubella and congenital rubella syndrome (CRS) from the Region by 2010. The elimination of rubella and CRS in the Americas has been defined as the successful interruption of endemic transmission of rubella virus in all countries of the Region without the occurrence of CRS cases associated with endemic transmission (*77*). As of July 2004, approximately 99% of new birth cohorts in the Americas have had access to the combination measles, mumps, and rubella vaccine (MMR) (*78*). In addition, targeted vaccination of adolescents and adults is a strategy designed to rapidly reduce the population susceptible to rubella infection, ultimately eliminating rubella virus transmission and congenital rubella syndrome.

Between 1998 and July 2004, Costa Rica, Ecuador, El Salvador, Honduras, Mexico, and the countries of the English-speaking Caribbean conducted adult vaccination campaigns targeting women and men. Campaigns in Brazil and Chile targeted only women of childbearing age. During the campaign, coverage in the Caribbean reached 80%; coverage rates in the other countries reached >95% (*78*).

To achieve the regional elimination goals, the remaining countries in the Region should conduct adult vaccination campaigns by 2007. The age group to be vaccinated should be determined based on an analysis of the likely susceptibility of adults. This would depend on the year of introduction of the MMR vaccine in the national schedule, the extent of follow-up MR or MMR vaccination campaigns to maintain measles elimination, and the rubella epidemiology in the country. Countries that have conducted mass vaccination campaigns only in women should determine the extent of the virus transmission and susceptibility in men, and develop appropriate strategies to reduce the number of rubella-susceptible men.

Substantial evidence has accumulated from many studies, including recent studies in Brazil and Costa Rica, that indicates that there is no identifiable link between vaccinating pregnant women and their giving birth to a child with CRS (79). Therefore, there is no reason to modify the current approach of vaccinating all women of childbearing age during campaigns.

MENINGOCOCCAL VACCINATION IN ADULTS

Although relatively uncommon, meningococcal disease is devastating when it occurs in epidemics and tragic to individual families when endemic. The highest incidence is in the first year of life, but another peak occurs in adolescence. Polysaccharide vaccines have been available for some time, and have been effective for time-limited protection. Recently, protein-conjugated meningococcal polysaccharide vaccines have been developed against four of the five major serogroups of the organism: A, C, W-135, and Y (80). The conjugated vaccines induce high titers of bactericidal antibodies, immunological memory, and also interfere with pharyngeal carriage. The latter property results in herd immunity and reduction of disease in the unvaccinated.

Application of a monovalent Group C vaccine has dramatically reduced disease in the United Kingdom (81), and the quadrivalent vaccine has just been recommended for American preadolescents and adolescents.

Group B vaccines have been difficult to develop, but several countries using regional vaccines based on outer-membrane proteins have achieved some success in controlling group B meningococcal disease epidemics (82).

PERTUSSIS VACCINATION IN ADULTS

Pertussis cases declined significantly in the Americas during the 1980s (Figure 1), yet several cases still occur annually, and there also are periodic case peaks. Although improved diagnosis undoubtedly plays a role in detecting cases, it appears that pertussis incidence has increased in adolescents and adults, even in countries where pediatric vaccination is strong. This primarily appears to be the result of waning immunity from vaccine, despite 70%–90% protection against severe disease conferred by a four-dose primary series with whole-cell vaccine. Pertussis disease in older individuals is not only frequent and disabling for the patient, but also serves as a source of infection for non-immunized infants, with associated high case-fatality rates.

Recently, Td booster vaccines containing acellular pertussis antigens (Tdap) have been licensed for use in adolescents and adults in the United States and Canada. In 2005, the United States recommended routine use of a single dose of Tdap for adults 19–64 years of age, to replace the next booster dose of tetanus and diphtheria toxoids vaccine (Td) for adults who have close contact with infants <12 months of age and for health-care personnel when feasible.

These contain a lower dose of the acellular pertussis component than the vaccines licensed and used for children and infants aged <7 years. Trials on acellular pertussis vaccine have shown variable efficacies and it is not yet known if the duration of protection and effectiveness of acellular pertussis is comparable with whole-cell pertussis vaccines (83).

Considering the effectiveness and lower prices of whole-cell pertussis vaccines, PAHO's Technical Advisory Group (TAG) and the World Health Organization recommend that when resources are limited and whole-cell vaccine is well-accepted by the population, these should be the vaccines of choice. In countries where high reactogenicity of whole-cell vaccine is an impediment for achieving high coverages, acellular pertussis vaccines may be used for booster doses (84, 85).

YELLOW FEVER VACCINATION IN ADULTS

Urban and jungle yellow fever are epidemiologically distinguishable from one another if one considers transmission cycles; however, clinically and etiologically they are identical. The urban yellow fever cycle is characterized by circulation of virus among susceptible humans transmitted from infected to susceptible persons by *Aedes aegypti* mosquitoes, which breed in domestic and peridomestic containers.

In the jungle cycle, the virus circulates among nonhuman primates and eventually among susceptible marsupials; transmission occurs through jungle-species mosquitoes, such as those from the genera *Haemagogus* and *Sabethes*. Humans are infected in jungle areas, entering the jungle transmission cycle. An enzootic area is a region in which there is confirmed viral circulation and ecologic conditions maintain viral transmission in the jungle cycle.

Urban yellow fever can be prevented by vaccinating human populations at risk for infection and/or by suppressing populations of *Ae. aegypti* mosquitoes so that they no longer perpetuate infection. Jungle yellow fever can most effectively be prevented by vaccination of human populations at risk for exposure.

In 2003, 242 confirmed cases of yellow fever were reported in the Americas, with a case-fatality rate of 44%. The number of confirmed cases was three times higher than that reported in 2002. Over 80% of the cases in these years were related to outbreaks in Brazil, Colombia, Venezuela, and Peru. The outbreaks in Colombia, Venezuela, and Peru occurred in traditionally enzootic areas; the outbreak in Brazil occurred in an area that was not considered enzootic, and thus was not the object of vaccination activities. In 2004, 118 cases were reported, with a 49% case-fatality. Most cases were associated with yellow fever outbreaks reported in Bolivia, Colombia, and Peru. Isolated cases have also been identified in Brazil and Venezuela (Figure 3) (*78*).

Yellow fever vaccine is a live, attenuated virus, which is considered to be one of the safest and most effective live virus vaccines ever developed. All current vaccines are made from the 17D yellow fever virus strain (17D-204 lineage and 17DD lineage). The virus is grown in chick embryos inoculated with a seed virus of a fixed passage level. Reactions to 17D yellow fever vaccine are typically mild, involving such symptoms as headaches, myalgia, and low-grade fevers.

PAHO's Technical Advisory Group (TAG) recommends that countries that have enzootic areas vaccinate residents in those areas against yellow fever and gradually introduce the vaccine into their routine immunization schedule (*78*). All children aged 12 months and older should be vaccinated in these areas, reaching a minimum coverage of 95%. In addition, residents of areas where migrations to enzootic areas originate should also be vaccinated (*86*). Because attack rates are higher in travelers and professionals entering viral circulation areas, vaccination targeting populations traveling or migrating to enzootic areas is important. In non-enzootic areas, the vaccine should be administered to travelers entering enzootic areas.

International Health Regulations require revaccination at intervals of 10 years (*86*). Revaccination can boost antibody titer; however, evidence from multiple studies (*87–90*) demonstrates that yellow fever vaccine immunity persists for 30–35 years and probably for life.

The vaccine is contraindicated in infants <6 months, since they are likely to be more susceptible to the serious adverse reaction of neuotropic disease associated with yellow fever vaccine. Yellow fever vaccine also should not be administered to individuals with a history of hypersensitivity to chicken eggs and their derivatives, or to immunosuppressed individuals.

FIGURE 3. Distribution of cases and deaths due to jungle yellow fever
in enzootic areas, Region of the Americas, 1999–2004.

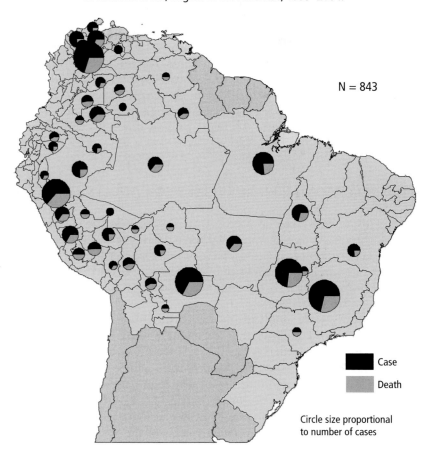

N = 843

■ Case

▓ Death

Circle size proportional
to number of cases

Source: Immunization Unit, Pan American Health Organization.

Because the safety of yellow fever vaccination during pregnancy has not yet been established, the vaccine should only be administered to pregnant women if they must travel to an endemic area and if an increased risk for exposure exists. There are no reports of adverse events or transmission of the 17D vaccine viruses from nursing mother to infant; however, since it is not known whether this vaccine is excreted in human milk, vaccination of nursing mothers should be avoided as a precautionary measure.

In recent years, some serious adverse reactions associated with the vaccine have been reported in previously healthy individuals in the United

States (9 cases), Brazil (4 cases), and Australia, Colombia, France, Switzerland, and the United Kingdom (1 case each). These involved viscerotropic disease associated with yellow fever vaccine, which is similar to fulminant yellow fever caused by wild-type yellow fever virus. Thus, both the 17DD and 17D-204 yellow fever vaccines must be considered as a possible, but rare, cause of severe adverse events. It is impossible to have an accurate measure of the incidence of this rare vaccine-associated viscerotropic disease due to the lack of adequate prospective data. However, crude estimates of the reported frequency range from 0.09 per 1 million doses distributed in Brazil to 2.5 per 1 million doses distributed in the United States (*86, 91*).

HUMAN PAPILLOMAVIRUS VACCINES FOR ADULTS

In 2006, HPV vaccine was licensed for the first time in the United States: quadrivalent vaccine is recommended for women aged 9–26 years. Other countries may soon license these vaccines and consider the vaccination of boys. Major effects on the incidence of cervical cancer are expected, but as happened with hepatitis B vaccination, effects will not be conclusively demonstrated for some years.

A cost-effectiveness analysis modeled the introduction of vaccine against HPV-16 and HPV-18 into vaccination programs in the United States (*92*). Vaccination of 12-year-old girls would reduce cervical cancer cases by 61.8%, with a cost-effectiveness ratio of US$ 14,583 per QALY. The study found that including male participants in a vaccine program would further reduce cervical cancer cases by 2.2%, but the measure was not cost-effective compared to female-only vaccination.

Another study evaluated cost-effectiveness of different cancer prevention policies, including vaccination, cytologic screening at various ages, and combined vaccination and screening. Assuming 90% vaccine effectiveness, the most cost-effective strategy was the combination of vaccination at age 12 years with triennial conventional cytologic screening beginning at age 25 years, which resulted in an incremental cost-effectiveness ratio of less than US$ 60,000 per QALY (*93*).

ADULT VACCINATION AGAINST SEXUALLY TRANSMITTED INFECTIONS

Experimental vaccines against herpes simplex type 2 have demonstrated definite but limited efficacy. Women who are seronegative to type 1 herpes simplex virus are the main beneficiaries, possibly because naturally acquired immunity to type 1 also confers protection (94). If phase 3 trials yield good results, an HSV vaccine may also be incorporated into pre-adolescent vaccination.

A vaccine against HIV is, of course, high priority. Once available it most likely will be offered to adolescents and adults.

VACCINES AGAINST CONGENITAL INFECTIONS

Rubella vaccine already offers protection against a congenitally acquired infection. Two other infections that are prevalent and that threaten the fetus are cytomegalovirus (CMV) and parvovirus B19. The former causes deafness and mental retardation; the latter causes fetal hydrops and still-birth. Several CMV vaccines are in clinical trial (95). Parvovirus B19 vaccine development is at an earlier stage (96).

VACCINES AGAINST HERPES ZOSTER

Cellular immunity to varicella decreases with age, allowing recrudes-cence of the virus in the form of herpes zoster, which is often painful and debilitating. Booster vaccination with the live varicella vaccine appears to restore that immunity. A large clinical trial of vaccination to prevent zoster will soon be reported (97).

WHEN TO VACCINATE ADOLESCENTS

Clearly, many vaccines are needed for adolescents, and fortunately, many new vaccines are in the pipeline. For many of the diseases these vaccines are meant to protect against, infection starts in adolescence, which makes it necessary to vaccinate before adolescence. Thus, vaccination of adolescents at ages 11–13 years, or after grade six, is likely to become the standard.

SUMMARY

As vaccination progresses into the 21st century, the trend is to expand from the traditional, standard pediatric vaccination to vaccination of all age groups. Adolescents will need booster vaccinations using several anti-gens to protect them during adult life, as well as new vaccinations against sexually transmitted infections and infections occurring in pregnancy. Adults later in life will need influenza and pneumococcal vaccines, and perhaps vaccination against zoster also.

References

1. Centers for Disease Control and Prevention. Prevention and Control of Influenza: Recommendations of the Advisory Committee on Immunization Practices (ACIP). *MMWR* 2005;54(RR08):1–40.
2. Izurieta HS, Thompson WW, Kramarz P, et al. Influenza and the rates of hospitalization for respiratory disease among infants and young children. *N Engl J Med* 2000;342:232–239.
3. Neuzil KM, Wright PF, Mitchel EF Jr., et al. The burden of influenza illness in children with asthma and other chronic medical conditions. *J Pediatr* 2000; 137:856–864.
4. Simonsen L, Clarke MJ, Schonberger LB, Arden NH, Cox NJ, Fukuda K. Pandemic versus epidemic influenza mortality: a pattern of changing age distribution. *J Infect Dis* 1998;178:53-60.
5. Thompson WW, Shay DK, Weintraub E, et al. Mortality associated with influenza and respiratory syncytial virus in the United States. *JAMA* 2003;289: 179–186.
6. La Montagne JR, Noble GR, Quinnan GV, et al. Summary of clinical trials of inactivated influenza vaccine—1978. *Rev Infect Dis* 1983;5:723–736.
7. Hirota Y, Kaji M, Ide S, et al. Antibody efficacy as a keen index to evaluate influenza vaccine effectiveness. *Vaccine* 1997;15:962–967.
8. Wilde JA, McMillan JA, Serwint J, Butta J, O'Riordan MA, Steinhoff MC. Effectiveness of influenza vaccine in health care professionals: a randomized trial. *JAMA* 1999;281:908–913.
9. Bridges CB, Thompson WW, Meltzer MI, et al. Effectiveness and cost-benefit of influenza vaccination of healthy working adults: a randomized controlled trial. *JAMA* 2000;284:1655–1663.
10. Demicheli V, Jefferson T, Rivetti D, Deeks J. Prevention and early treatment of influenza in healthy adults. *Vaccine* 2000;18:957–1030.
11. Smith JW, Pollard R. Vaccination against influenza: a five-year study in the Post Office. *J Hyg* (Lond) 1979;83:157–170.
12. McElhaney JE, Beattie BL, Devine R, et al. Age-related decline in interleukin 2 production in response to influenza vaccine. *J Am Geriatr Soc* 1990;38:652–658.
13. Dorrell L, Hassan I, Marshall S, et al. Clinical and serological responses to an inactivated influenza vaccine in adults with HIV infection, diabetes, obstructive airways disease, elderly adults and healthy volunteers. *Int J STD AIDS* 1997;8:776–779.
14. Govaert TM, Thijs CT, Masurel N, et al. The efficacy of influenza vaccination in elderly individuals. A randomized double-blind placebo-controlled trial. *JAMA* 1994;272:1661–1665.
15. Nichol KL, Wuorenma J, von Sternberg T. Benefits of influenza vaccination for low-, intermediate-, and high-risk senior citizens. *Arch Intern Med* 1998;158: 1769–1776.
16. Mullooly JP, Bennett MD, Hornbrook MC, et al. Influenza vaccination programs for elderly persons: cost-effectiveness in a health maintenance organization. *Ann Intern Med* 1994;121:947–952.
17. Patriarca PA, Weber JA, Parker RA, et al. Efficacy of influenza vaccine in nursing homes: reduction in illness and complications during an influenza A (H3N2) epidemic. *JAMA* 1985;253:1136–1139.

18. Nordin J, Mullooly J, Poblete S, et al. Influenza vaccine effectiveness in preventing hospitalizations and deaths in persons 65 years or older in Minnesota, New York, and Oregon: data from 3 health plans. *J Infect Dis* 2001;184:665–670.
19. Hak E, Nordin J, Wei F, et al. Influence of high-risk medical conditions on the effectiveness of influenza vaccination among elderly members of 3 large managed-care organizations. *Clin Infect Dis* 2002;35:370–377.
20. Nichol KL, Nordin J, Mullooly J, Lask R, Fillbrandt K, Iwane M. Influenza vaccination and reduction in hospitalizations for cardiac disease and stroke among the elderly. *N Engl J Med* 2003 Apr 3;348(14):1322–1332.
21. Monto AS, Hornbuckle K, Ohmit SE. Influenza vaccine effectiveness among elderly nursing home residents: a cohort study. *Am J Epidemiol* 2001;154: 155–160.
22. Riddiough MA, Sisk JE, Bell JC. Influenza vaccination. *JAMA* 1983;249: 3189–3195.
23. Nichol KL, Lind A, Margolis KL, et al. Effectiveness of vaccination against influenza in healthy, working adults. *N Engl J Med* 1995;333:889–893.
24. Campbell DS, Rumley MH. Cost-effectiveness of the influenza vaccine in a healthy, working-age population. *J Occup Environ Med* 1997;39:408–414.
25. Mixeu MA, Vespa GNR, Forleo-Neto E, Toniolo-Neto J, Alves PM. Impact of influenza vaccination on civilian aircrew illness and absenteeism. *Aviat Space Environ Med* 2002;73:876–880.
26. Nichol KL. Cost-benefit analysis of a strategy to vaccinate healthy working adults against influenza. *Arch Intern Med* 2001;161:749–759.
27. Office of Technology Assessment. Cost effectiveness of influenza vaccination. Washington, DC: US Congress, 1981.
28. Cate TR, Couch RB, Parker D, Baxter B. Reactogenicity, immunogenicity, and antibody persistence in adults given inactivated influenza virus vaccines— 1978. *Rev Infect Dis* 1983;5:737–747.
29. Kunzel W, Glathe H, Engelmann H, Van Hoecke C. Kinetics of humoral antibody response to trivalent inactivated split influenza vaccine in subjects previously vaccinated or vaccinated for the first time. *Vaccine* 1996;14:1108–1110.
30. Brokstad KA, Cox RJ, Olofsson J, et al. Parenteral influenza vaccination induces a rapid systemic and local immune response. *J Infect Dis* 1995;171:198–203.
31. Gross PA, Russo C, Dran S, et al. Time to earliest peak serum antibody response to influenza vaccine in the elderly. *Clin Diagn Lab Immunol* 1997;4:491–492.
32. Potter J, Stott DJ, Roberts MA, et al. Influenza vaccination of health care workers in long-term-care hospitals reduces the mortality of elderly patients. *J Infect Dis* 1997;175:1–6.
33. Carman WF, Elder AG, Wallace LA, et al. Effects of influenza vaccination of health-care workers on mortality of elderly people in long-term care: a randomised controlled trial. *Lancet* 2000;355:93–97.
34. Neuzil KM, Mellen BG, Wright PF, Mitchel EF, Griffin MR. Effect of influenza on hospitalizations, outpatient visits, and courses of antibiotics in children. *N Engl J Med* 2000;342:225–231.
35. Feery BJ, Cheyne IM, Hampson AW, Atkinson MI. Antibody response to one and two doses of influenza virus subunit vaccine. *Med J Aust* 1976;1:186–89.
36. Levine M, Beattie BL, McLean DM. Comparison of one- and two-dose regimens of influenza vaccine for elderly men. *CMAJ* 1987;137:722–726.

37. Poland GA, Borrud A, Jacobson RM, et al. Determination of deltoid fat pad thickness: implications for needle length in adult immunization. *JAMA* 1997; 277:1709–1711.
38. Centers for Disease Control and Prevention (CDC). Prevention of Pneumococcal Disease: Recommendations of the Advisory Committee on Immunization Practices (ACIP). *MMWR* 1997;46(RR-08):1–24.
39. Klein DL, Ellis RW. Conjugate vaccines against *Streptococcus pneumoniae*. In: Levine MM, Woodrow GC, Kaper JB, Cobon, GS, eds. *New generation vaccines*. 2nd ed., rev. New York, NY: Marcel Dekker, Inc., 1997:503–525.
40. Mbelle N, Huebner RE, Wasas AD, Kimura A, Chang I, Klugman K. Immunogenicity and impact on nasopharyngeal carriage of a nonavalent pneumococcal conjugate vaccine. *J Infect Dis* 1999;180:1171–1176.
41. Black S, Shinefield H, Fireman B, et al. Efficacy, safety and immunogenicity of heptavalent pneumococcal conjugate vaccine in children. *Pediatr Infect Dis J* 2000;19:187–195.
42. Centers for Disease Control and Prevention (CDC). Active Bacterial Core Surveillance (ABCs) Report, Emerging Infections Program Network (EIP), *Streptococcus pneumoniae*, 1998. Atlanta, GA: US Department of Health and Human Services, CDC, 1999. Available at http://www.cdc.gov/ncidod/dbmd/abcs/spneu98.pdf. Accessed August 4, 2000.
43. Istre GR, Tarpay M, Anderson M, Pryor A, Welch D, Pneumococcus Study Group. Invasive disease due to *Streptococcus pneumoniae* in an area with a high rate of relative penicillin resistance. *J Infect Dis* 1987;156:732–735.
44. Breiman RF, Spika JS, Navarro VJ, Darden PM, Darby CP. Pneumococcal bacteremia in Charleston County, South Carolina: a decade later. *Arch Intern Med* 1990;150:1401–1405.
45. Bennett NM, Buffington J, LaForce FM. Pneumococcal bacteremia in Monroe County, New York. *Am J Public Health* 1992;82:1513–1516.
46. Afessa B, Greaves WL, Frederick WR. Pneumococcal bacteremia in adults: a 14-year experience in an inner-city university hospital. *Clin Infect Dis* 1995;21: 345–351.
47. Hook EW, Horton CA, Schaberg DR. Failure of intensive care unit support to influence mortality from pneumococcal bacteremia. *JAMA* 1983;249:1055–1057.
48. Plouffe JF, Breiman RF, Facklam RR, Franklin County Pneumonia Study Group. Bacteremia with *Streptococcus pneumoniae* in adults—implications for therapy and prevention. *JAMA* 1996;275:194–198.
49. Mufson MA, Krause HE, Schiffman G, Hughey DF. Pneumococcal antibody levels one decade after immunization of healthy adults. *Am J Med Sci* 1987;293: 279–289.
50. Minor DR, Schiffman G, McIntosh LS. Response of patients with Hodgkin's disease to pneumococcal vaccine. *Ann Intern Med* 1979;90:887–892.
51. Mufson MA, Krause HE, Schiffman G. Long-term persistence of antibody following immunization with pneumococcal polysaccharide vaccine. *Proc Soc Exp Biol Med* 1983;173:270–275.
52. Vella PP, McLean AA, Woodhour AF, Weibel RE, Hilleman MR. Persistence of pneumococcal antibodies in human subjects following vaccination. *Proc Soc Exp Biol Med* 1980;164:435–438.
53. Hilleman MR, Carlson AJ, McLean AA, Vella PP, Weibel RE, Woodhour AF. Streptococcus pneumoniae polysaccharide vaccine: age and dose responses,

safety, persistence of antibody, revaccination, and simultaneous administration of pneumococcal and influenza vaccines. *Rev Infect Dis* 1981;3(suppl):S31–S42.

54. Kraus C, Fischer S, Ansorg R, Hüttemann U. Pneumococcal antibodies (IgG, IgM) in patients with chronic obstructive lung disease 3 years after pneumococcal vaccination. *Med Microbiol Immunol* 1985;174:51–58.

55. Fine MJ, Smith MA, Carson CA, et al. Efficacy of pneumococcal vaccination in adults: a meta-analysis of randomized controlled trials. *Arch Intern Med* 1994; 154:2666–2677.

56. Shapiro ED, Berg AT, Austrian R, et al. The protective efficacy of polyvalent pneumococcal polysaccharide vaccine. *N Engl J Med* 1991;325:1453–1460.

57. Jackson LA, Neuzil KM, Yu O, Benson P, Barlow WE, Adams AL, Hanson CA, Mahoney LD, Shay DK, Thompson WW; Vaccine Safety Datalink. Effectiveness of pneumococcal polysaccharide vaccine in older adults. *N Engl J Med* 2003 May 1;348(18):1747–1755.

58. Lexau CA, Lynfield R, Danila R, Pilishvili T, Facklam R, Farley MM, Harrison LH, Schaffner W, Reingold A, Bennett NM, Hadler J, Cieslak PR, Whitney CG; Active Bacterial Core Surveillance Team. Changing epidemiology of invasive pneumococcal disease among older adults in the era of pediatric pneumococcal conjugate vaccine. *JAMA* 2005 Oct 26;294(16):2043–2051.

59. Melegaro A, Edmunds WJ. The 23-valent pneumococcal polysaccharide vaccine. Part II. A cost-effectiveness analysis for invasive disease in the elderly in England and Wales. *Eur J Epidemiol* 2004;19(4):365–375.

60. Kelly H, Attia J, Andrews R, Heller RF. The number needed to vaccinate (NNV) and population extensions of the NNV: comparison of influenza and pneumococcal vaccine programmes for people aged 65 years and over. *Vaccine* 2004 Jun 2;22(17–18):2192–2198.

61. Postma MJ, Heijnen ML, Beutels P, Jager JC. Pharmacoeconomics of elderly vaccination against invasive pneumococcal infections: cost-effectiveness analyses and implications for The Netherlands. *Expert Rev Vaccines* 2003 Aug; 2(4):477–482.

62. Sisk JE, Whang W, Butler JC, Sneller VP, Whitney CG. Cost-effectiveness of vaccination against invasive pneumococcal disease among people 50 through 64 years of age: role of comorbid conditions and race. *Ann Intern Med* 2003 Jun 17;138(12):960–968.

63. Pepper PV, Owens DK. Cost-effectiveness of the pneumococcal vaccine in healthy younger adults. *Med Decis Making* 2002 Sep-Oct;22(5 suppl):S45–S57.

64. Mufson MA, Hughey DF, Turner CE, Schiffman G. Revaccination with pneumococcal vaccine of elderly persons 6 years after primary vaccination. *Vaccine* 1991;9:403–407.

65. Torling J, Hedlund J, Konradsen HB, Ortqvist A. Revaccination with the 23-valent pneumococcal polysaccharide vaccine in middle-aged and elderly persons previously treated for pneumonia. *Vaccine* 2003 Dec 8;22(1):96–103.

66. Lackner TE, G Hamilton R, J Hill J, Davey C, Guay DR. Pneumococcal polysaccharide revaccination: immunoglobulin g seroconversion, persistence, and safety in frail, chronically ill older subjects. *J Am Geriatr Soc* 2003 Feb;51(2): 240–245.

67. Butler JC, Breiman RF, Campbell JF, Lipman HB, Broome CV, Facklam RR. Pneumococcal polysaccharide vaccine efficacy: an evaluation of current recommendations. *JAMA* 1993;270:1826–1831.

68. Centers for Disease Control and Prevention (CDC).Update on Adult Immunization Recommendations of the Immunization Practices Advisory Committee (ACIP). *MMWR* 1991;40(RR12):1–52.
69. Crossley K, Irvine P, Warren JB, Lee BK, Mead K. Tetanus and diphtheria immunity in urban Minnesota adults. *JAMA* 1979;242:2298–3000.
70. Ruben FL, Nagel J, Fireman P. Antitoxin responses in the elderly to tetanus-diphtheria (Td) immunization. *Am J Epidemiol* 1978;108:145–149.
71. Weiss BP, Strassburg MA, Feeley JC. Tetanus and diphtheria immunity in an elderly population in Los Angeles County. *Am J Public Health* 1983;73:802–804.
72. Koblin BA, Townsend TR. Immunity to diphtheria and tetanus in inner-city women of childbearing age. *Am J Public Health* 1989;79:1297–1298.
73. Robertson SE, Featherstone DA, Gacic DM, Hersh BS. Rubella and congenital rubella syndrome: global update. *Rev Panam Salud Publica* 2003;14:306–315.
74. Centers for Disease Control and Prevention (CDC). Elimination of rubella and congenital rubella syndrome—United States, 1969-2004. *MMWR* 2005 Mar 25; 54(11):279–282.
75. Davidkin I, Peltola H, Leinikki P. Epidemiology of rubella in Finland. *Euro Surveill* 2004 Apr 1;9(4).
76. Peltola H, Heinonen OP, Valle M, Paunio M, Virtanen M, Karanko V, Cantell K. The elimination of indigenous measles, mumps, and rubella from Finland by a 12-year, two-dose vaccination program. *N Engl J Med* 1994 Nov 24;331 (21):1397–1402.
77. Castillo-Solorzano C, Andrus JK. Rubella elimination and improving health care for women. *Emerg Infect Dis* 2004 Nov;10(11):2017–2021.
78. Pan-American Health Organization. XVI Technical Advisory Group (TAG) Meeting on Vaccine Preventable-Diseases, 2004. Final report of the XVI TAG Meeting on Vaccine Preventable-Diseases of the Pan American Health Organization, held in Mexico City, Mexico, November 3–5, 2004. Available at: http://www.paho.org/English/AD/FCH/IM/TAG16_FinalReport_2004. pdf.
79. Soares R, Toscano CM, Siqueira MM, Will RM, Fagundes MF, Rodrigues RCM, Barbosa TC, Sá GRS, Figueiredo MF, Morhdieck R, Castillo-Solorzano C, Maia MLS, Camacho LA, Luna E. Follow-up study of women who were unknowingly pregnant and vaccinated against rubella in Brazil, 2001–2002. Oral presentation at the XVI Meeting of the Pan American Technical Advisory Group on Vaccine Preventable Diseases. Mexico City, Mexico. November, 2004.
80. Pichichero M, Casey J, Blatter M, et al. Comparative trial of the safety and immunogenicity of quadrivalent (A, C, Y, W-135) meningococcal polysaccharide-diphtheria conjugate vaccine versus quadrivalent polysaccharide vaccine in two- to ten-year-old children. *Pediatr Infect Dis J* 2005;24:57–62.
81. Snape MD, Pollard AJ. Meningococcal polysaccharide-protein conjugate vaccines. *Lancet Infect Dis* 2005;5:21–30.
82. Ameratunga S, Macmillan A, Stewart J, Scott D, Mulholland K, Crengle S. Evaluating the post-licensure effectiveness of a group B meningococcal vaccine in New Zealand: a multi-faceted strategy. *Vaccine* 2005;23:2231–2234.
83. Decker MD, Bogaert HH. Combination vaccines. In: Plotkin SA, Orenstein WA, eds. *Vaccines*, 4th ed. Philadelphia: W.B. Saunders Co., 2004:825–854.
84. Pan American Health Organization. *Final report (conclusions and recommendations).* XII Meeting of the Technical Advisory Group (TAG) on Vaccine-preventable Diseases. Washington, DC: PAHO; 1997.

85. World Health Organization. Pertussis vaccines. *Wkly Epidemiol Rec* 2005;80(4): 31–39.
86. Pan American Health Organization. Control of Yellow Fever: Field Guide. Scientific and Technical Publication No. 603. Washington, DC: PAHO, 2005.
87. Groot H, Ribeiro RB. Neutralizing and haemagglutination-inhibiting antibodies to yellow fever 17 years after vaccination with 17D vaccine. *Bull WHO* 1962;27:669–707.
88. Rosenzweig EC, Babione RW, Wisseman CL Jr. Immunological studies with group B arthropod-borne viruses. IV. Persistence of yellow fever antibodies following vaccination with 17D strain yellow fever vaccine. *Am J Trop Med Hyg* 1963;12:230–235.
89. Poland JD, Calisher CH, Monath TP, Downs WG, Murphy K. Persistence of neutralizing antibody 30–35 years after immunization with 17D yellow fever vaccine. *Bull WHO* 1981;59:895–900.
90. Niedrig M, Lademann M, Emmerich P, Lafrenz M. Assessment of IgG antibodies against yellow fever virus after vaccination with 17D by different assays: neutralization test, haemagglutination inhibition test, immunofluorescence assay and ELISA. *Trop Med Int Health* 1999;4:867–871.
91. Centers for Disease Control and Prevention (CDC). Yellow Fever Vaccine Recommendations of the Advisory Committee on Immunization Practices (ACIP), 2002. *MMWR* November 8, 2002;51(RR17):1–10.
92. Taira AV, Neukermans CP, Sanders GD. Evaluating human papillomavirus vaccination programs. *Emerg Infect Dis* 2004 Nov;10(11):1915–1923.
93. Goldie SJ, Kohli M, Grima D, Weinstein MC, Wright TC, Bosch FX, Franco E. Projected clinical benefits and cost-effectiveness of a human papillomavirus 16/18 vaccine. *J Natl Cancer Inst* 2004 Apr 21;96(8):604–615.
94. Stanberry LR, Spruance SL, Cunningham AL, et al. Glycoprotein-D-adjuvant vaccine to prevent genital herpes. *N Engl J Med* 2002;347:1652–1661.
95. Arvin AM, Fast P, Myers M, Plotkin SA, Rabinovich R. Vaccine development to prevent cytomegalovirus disease: report from the National Vaccine Advisory Committee. *Clin Infect Dis* 2000;39:233–239.
96. Ballou WR, Reed JL, Noble W, Young NS, Koenig S, Safety and immunogenicity of a recombinant parvovirus B19 vaccine formulated with MF59C.1. *J Infect Dis* 2003;187:675–678.
97. Oxman MN. Immunization to reduce the frequency and severity of herpes zoster and its complications. *Neurology* 1995;45:S41–S46.

COMBINATION VACCINES FOR CHILDHOOD IMMUNIZATION

José Ignacio Santos, MD, MSc[1] and Orin Levine, PhD[2]

INTRODUCTION

Vaccination is one of the most valuable and cost-effective strategies available to medicine in the battle to prevent and control infectious diseases. It is considered to be one of the ten greatest public health achievements of the 20th century *(1)*. In the Americas, vaccination has brought about the eradication of smallpox in 1970 and of polio in 1991; the interruption of indigenous measles transmission in 2002; and the lowest numbers of reported cases of congenital rubella syndrome (CRS) and neonatal tetanus at the onset of the 21st century *(1, 2)*.

Over the last four decades, important new and improved vaccines to prevent childhood diseases have been developed; more are in the pipeline. As the number of vaccine-preventable diseases increases, so does the number of injections a child must receive to be fully protected. In 1999, the Recommended Childhood Immunization Schedule in the United States included 10 different vaccines—hepatitis B (Hep B); diphtheria, pertussis, and tetanus (DPT); *Haemophilus influenzae* type b (Hib); injectable polio vaccine (IPV) or oral polio vaccine (OPV); measles, mumps, and rubella (MMR); and varicella—which required a minimum of 13 injections to immunize a child from birth to age 6 years *(3)*. By 2005, the United States childhood immunization schedule *(4)* recommended the inclusion of two additional vaccines: the conjugated pneumococcal vaccine (PCV) and the influenza vaccine. At this juncture, OPV was replaced with IPV, and diph-

[1] General Director, Hospital Infantil de México Federico Gómez, México D.F.
[2] Executive Director, Global Alliance for Vaccines and Immunization's PneumoADIP, Johns Hopkins Bloomberg School of Public Health.

theria, tetanus, and whole-cell pertussis (DTwP) was replaced with diphtheria, tetanus, and acellular pertussis (DtaP). Thus, the current United States childhood vaccination schedule now requires between 18 and 21 separate injections before a child enters school and as many as 5 separate injections in a single doctor's office visit. Most Latin American countries, on the other hand, follow a schedule that differs both in the number and the type of vaccines—10 vaccines, including BCG at birth; OPV, DTwP, Hib, and Hep B at 2, 4, and 6 months; and MMR at 12 months, require between 6 and 7 injections before school entry and as many as 2 separate injections during a single clinic visit (5).

Judging by recent vaccine coverage levels in the United States and the rest of the Region of the Americas, the number of injections required at this time does not appear to deter parents from vaccinating their children. There are two potential threats to the future of immunization programs, however. As new vaccines are introduced, requiring more injections, the acceptance threshold may begin to decline.

Equally worrisome is the fact that, as specific diseases preventable by immunization are contained, the public's perception of disease risk and vaccine benefit for a disease that is no longer common may negatively affect the acceptance of numerous injections. A way to reduce the number of injections without reducing the number of diseases for which a child receives protection is to use combination vaccines (6–9).

COMBINATION VACCINES

Combination vaccines contain multiple antigens combined into a single preparation by the manufacturer or by the health-care worker, providing protection against multiple diseases. DTP is an excellent example of a combination vaccine, which protects against diphtheria, tetanus, and pertussis. There also are combination vaccines that protect against multiple strains of an infection that cause the same disease (multivalent vaccines), such as the Sabin oral attenuated polio vaccine (OPV) and the injectable Salk inactivated polio vaccine (IPV), both of which protect against polio viruses 1, 2, and 3. And there are vaccines that protect against serotypes of the same organism, such as the currently licensed heptavalent conjugated pneumococcal vaccine (PNV), which protects against the seven serotypes of *Streptococcus pneumoniae*. Another example is the trivalent influenza vaccine, which is prepared yearly with three inactivated viruses, type A (H1N1), type A (H3N2), and type B.

The use of combination vaccines reduces the number of injections required to prevent specific diseases and, in so doing, reduces trauma and pain experienced by the recipient (9, 10). Other potential advantages or attributes of combination vaccines are that they: a) improve the timeliness of vaccination coverage, b) reduce costs associated with stockpiling and administering separate vaccines, c) reduce costs associated with extra health care visits that result from delayed vaccinations, and d) facilitate the integration of new vaccines into the childhood immunization schedule. Although the price of a new combination vaccine usually exceeds the total price of separate vaccines for the same diseases, the extra expense should be considered against the direct and indirect costs of extra injections, delayed or missed vaccinations, and additional handling and storage (11, 12).

PAST, PRESENT, AND FUTURE COMBINATION VACCINES

Combination vaccines have been available for more than half a century. The concept was put into practice in the United States in 1945, with the licensing and introduction of the trivalent influenza vaccine; a hexavalent pneumococcal polysaccharide vaccine followed in 1947. It wasn't until the licensing of the combination vaccine that included diphtheria and tetanus toxoids and whole-cell pertussis (DTwP) in 1948, however, that combination vaccines had widespread acceptance in routine vaccination practices of infants and children. Seven years later, the trivalent inactivated polio virus vaccine (IPV) was licensed and introduced. Then came the oral polio vaccine (OPV) in 1962 and the measles-mumps-rubella vaccine (MMR) in 1971.

More recently, additional combination vaccines have been licensed and introduced into the immunization schedule of children in the United States, including: diphtheria and tetanus toxoids and acellular pertussis vaccine (DTaP); DTwP-*Haemophilus influenzae* type b (Hib) vaccine (DTwP-Hib); DTaP-Hib; *Haemophilus influenzae* type b conjugate vaccine-hepatitis B vaccine; diphtheria-tetanus-acellular pertussis-hepatitis B-inactivated poliovirus vaccine; pneumococcal conjugate vaccine (which contains seven serotypes of *Streptococcus pneumoniae* conjugated); and the trivalent influenza vaccine (13–15). Combination vaccines recently introduced in Latin American countries include the DTwP-Hep B-Hib vaccine. This combination vaccine allowed Hep B and Hib vaccines to be introduced without adding new injections. Rubella and mumps vaccines also have been added to many country schedules by combining rubella and mumps antigens with the measles antigen (MR and MMR vaccines).

The great variety of available combination-vaccine options poses a challenge for the clinician who must keep current with new knowledge about the antigens in the combinations, let alone the commercial names. In the future, additional combination vaccines designed to protect against other diseases are likely to emerge. They will need to be tailored to regional needs wherever the prevalence and disease burden of known, emerging, or reemerging diseases may justify their manufacture. It should be kept in mind, however, that although most of the technology and infrastructure needed to manufacture these products resides in industrialized countries, these combination vaccines may not necessarily be a priority in the country of origin. WHO recognizes that, other than the United States and Canada, there are three Western Hemisphere countries that are capable of producing vaccines: Brazil (through the Oswaldo Cruz Foundation and the Butantan Institute), Cuba (through its Center for Genetic Engineering and Biotechnology, known for its Spanish acronym, CIGB), and Mexico (through the Mexican Laboratories for Biologicals and Reagents, known for its Spanish acronym, BIRMEX). All three are attempting to satisfy local needs.

IMMUNOGENICITY AND EFFICACY OF COMBINATION VACCINES

Combination vaccines differ from single-component vaccines in makeup and in how they are manufactured. Combining multiple antigens into one preparation requires the in vitro demonstration of chemical compatibility. In addition, clinical trials are needed to substantiate that there is no decrease in the safety of the combined vaccines or immunologic interference when different antigens and other components (such as adjuvants, stabilizers, and preservatives) are combined into one vaccine. Such interference could compromise the safety, immunogenicity, and efficacy of the combined vaccine. Chemical incompatibility or immunologic interference when different antigens are combined into one vaccine are difficult challenges to overcome. The carrier proteins of conjugate vaccines may suppress or increase the response of other preparations containing these. In a combination vaccine, the adjuvant should improve the response to at least one of the relevant antigen(s), without exerting a clinically significant detrimental effect on immune responses to any other antigen in the vaccine (16–18).

Because each combination vaccine is unique, existing guidelines often fail to provide sufficient information to overcome the inevitable problems encountered when developing and implementing potency tests. Another potential challenge in giving vaccines in combination is that it may not always be clear which component is responsible for a particular adverse event. Combination vaccines from different manufacturers may have different recommended dosage schedules, potentially increasing the confusion for the provider (19).

Since the licensing of the diphtheria, tetanus, whole-cell pertussis vaccine (DTwP) in 1948, its impact on childhood morbidity and mortality has been undisputed. Inclusion of DTwP in childhood immunization programs continues to have wide acceptance in routine immunization programs of infants and children throughout the world. However, the nature of the pertussis antigens in DTP may influence the immunogenicity and effectiveness of the vaccine.

In the clinical development of the DTwP-HB-Hib vaccine, studies were conducted in several countries to evaluate how incorporating Hib into a DTwP-HB tetravalent vaccine might improve protection and kinetics. This pentavalent vaccine proved to be highly immunogenic for all vaccine antigens and no interference was demonstrated for any of the antigens, including PRP/Hib. A very important, albeit unexpected, finding was that the kinetics response for the anti-HBs component was significantly improved in some combination vaccines (9, 20). The anti-HBs response reached a 95% seroprotection level ($\geq$10mIU/ml) after the second dose of the DTwP-HB and DTwP-HB-Hib vaccines. In contrast, when DTwP and HB were given separately, the seroprotection response level for the anti-HBs component after the second dose of both vaccines was only 66%. The tetravalent DTwP-HB vaccine mixed with Hib also induced protective antibody titers against diphtheria, tetanus, and *H. influenzae*, as well as high anti-pertussis titers. A study conducted in five Latin American countries and involving 400 subjects confirmed the immunogenicity and reactogenicity profile of the DTwP-HB-Hib pentavalent vaccine established earlier. In this study, the immunogenicity for the individual components of the pentavalent vaccine was 100% for tetanus, *Bordetella pertussis*, hepatitis B, and PRP (poly-ribitol-phosphate, the capsular polysaccharide of Hib) type b/Hib and 98% for diphtheria. Seroprotection levels and geometric mean titers (GMTs) were comparable with the group receiving separate injections of DTwP-HB + PRP-TT (20, 21).

The difficulty in interpreting the clinical significance of antibody interference with combination vaccines is highlighted by the experience of combinations containing acellular pertussis (aP) vaccines (22). Two trials in Europe found a significant difference in post-immunization levels of diphtheria antitoxin, depending on whether any pertussis antigens were present in the vaccine and what the nature of the antigens was (23). The addition of an efficacious whole-cell pertussis (wP) component to the diphtheria and tetanus vaccine increased the geometrical mean titer of diphtheria antitoxin in the recipients. The addition of aP or a poorly efficacious whole-cell pertussis vaccine produced lower geometrical mean titers of diphtheria, compared to diphtheria titers in tetanus vaccine. In a few children, the concentrations reached were considered non-protective, confirming the well known "adjuvant" effect of efficacious whole-cell pertussis vaccines.

Combinations of Hib vaccines with DTwP vaccines were generally not associated with significant diminutions in immunogenicity to the Hib or DTP components. When Hib vaccines were combined instead with some DTaP vaccines, however, significantly lower geometrical mean concentrations of anti-Hib capsular polysaccharide IgG were observed (24). The extent of this reduction is not the same for all DTaP-Hib combinations. DTaP-Hib combinations containing five-component acellular pertussis appear to show little, if any, such reduction (25–28). Most importantly, the clinical significance of the lower antibody concentrations remains unclear. Recently the United Kingdom has reported a rise in Hib cases in fully immunized children who received a DTaP-Hib preparation (29). While this observation clearly suggests that there may be clinical significance to these antibody differences, other factors, such as the accelerated three-dose regimen used in the country, may have also contributed to the observed rise in Hib cases as well.

Responding to a recent rise in the incidence of H. influenzae type b disease in the United Kingdom, researchers conducted a study to assess Hib antibody concentration and avidity before and after the administration of an Hib booster. The rise in incidence was temporarily linked to the use of diphtheria-tetanus-acellular pertussis combination vaccine (DTaP-Hib) during 1999–2002. Between 1999 and 2002, the United Kingdom used aP combination vaccine because of a shortage of whole-cell combination vaccine. Their data suggest that DTaP can interfere with normal antibody avidity maturation that occurs after priming with Hib vaccine, and may explain the increased incidence of H. influenzae type b after 1999 (30).

Dagan et al. (31) reported that infants who were given a diphtheria-tetanus-pertussis-polio-Hib vaccine in which the Hib component was conjugated to tetanus, simultaneously with a pneumococcal vaccine also conjugated to tetanus toxoid, had lower Hib PRP antibody concentrations than infants who had received pneumococcal vaccine conjugated to diphtheria toxoid. Furthermore, children who had received higher doses of pneumococcal tetanus conjugate had poorer responses.

Finally, a phase 2 randomized controlled trial conducted in two United Kingdom centers examined the immunogenicity and safety of two vaccines. It compared a combination 9-valent pneumococcal-group C meningococcal conjugate candidate vaccine (Pnc9-MenC) with a monovalent group C meningococcal conjugate vaccine (MenC) administered in addition to routine immunizations (diphtheria and tetanus toxoids and whole-cell pertussis [DTwP], Haemophilus influenzae type b [Hib] polyribosylribitol phosphate-tetanus toxoid protein conjugate, and oral polio vaccine) in infants aged 7 to 11 weeks. The results revealed that although the Pnc9-MenC vaccine administered to infants at ages 2, 3, and 4 months was safe and immunogenic for all contained pneumococcal serotypes, it demonstrated reduced group C meningococcal immunogenicity compared with the MenC vaccine. The immunogenicity of concomitantly administered Hib and DTwP vaccines also was diminished for group C meningococcus antigen. The authors conclude that the Pnc9-MenC vaccine as tested may not be a suitable replacement for individual MenC or pneumococcal glycoconjugate vaccines. More importantly, this study is unique in that it also evaluated the concomitant administration of seven vaccines, including three separate combination vaccines—DTwP, trivalent OPV, and Pnc9-MenC—underscoring the importance of assessing the immunogenicity of all co-administered vaccine antigens in prelicensure trials *(32)*.

In many cases, combination vaccines may give a lower but still protective immune response as compared to separate vaccines. Some vaccine efficacy studies have generated antibody levels that correlate with protection from disease. These "immunologic correlates" of protection are important because they allow us to assess the clinical significance of any immunologic interference.

REACTOGENICITY AND SAFETY OF COMBINATION VACCINES

There is substantial evidence that combining vaccines into one product does not increase the overall rate of clinically significant, temporally associated adverse events. With some combinations, such as DTaP, the rates are sometimes lower than when the component vaccines are given separately *(9, 15, 18)*. An important exception has been DTwP, the first combination vaccine licensed.

There have been long-standing concerns about the relative safety of the whole-cell pertussis component of this vaccine. The reactogenicity, temporally associated with the wP component of the DTwP vaccine, including redness and swelling at the site of injection, agitation, febrile seizures and hypotonic-hypo-responsive episodes, high fever, persistent crying, and a fear of rare, but serious, acute or chronic neurological events, led several countries to discontinue its inclusion in routine immunization programs and prompted the development of a new generation of pertussis vaccines, the acellular (aP) vaccines. It is important to mention that despite thorough investigations, the link suspected between wP vaccines and rare cases of permanent neurological damage has not been confirmed *(9, 35, 36)*. Schmitt et al. compared antibody responses in children receiving DTaP-HBV-IPV-Hib as one injection with children receiving the same antigens but with the Hib given at a different site. No difference was found in adverse events temporally associated with the different regimens *(34)*.

In 1998, a paper published in the *Lancet* was interpreted by anti-vaccine groups as showing a link between measles, mumps, and rubella vaccine and developmental disorder and bowel disease *(35)*, even though the authors said they had not proved such a link. Subsequent research has failed to find evidence for this link *(35, 36)*. The suggested mechanism behind the hypothesis was that combining antigens produced an unpredictable response. Some parents are concerned that multiple antigens may overload the infant's immune system. A recent review set in context the antigenic load from vaccines in comparison with that from the environment and emphasized the capacity of the immune system to respond effectively to numerous simultaneous antigens *(37)*. The tetravalent DTwP-HB vaccine mixed with Hib also induced protective antibody titers against diphtheria, tetanus, and *H. influenzae* and high anti-pertussis titers. Results involving 400 subjects did not reveal an increase in the reactogenicity with the addition of hepatitis B antigen to DTwP or the mixing of Hib with the DTwP-HB combination as compared to DTwP alone *(20, 21)*.

The preservative thimerosal plays a role in the heat inactivation of bacteria in the production of whole-cell pertussis vaccines and is present in DTwP and DTwP-Hib products. It is not present in some of the acellular pertussis products available such as DTaP and DTaP-Hib. A recent study has shown that the amount of mercury in the blood of children receiving thimerosal-containing vaccines is well below that potentially associated with any toxic effect, even when administered at 2 months of age *(38)*.

EXTRA DOSES AND INTERCHANGEABILITY OF COMBINATION VACCINE ANTIGENS

The Advisory Committee on Immunization Practices (ACIP), the American Academy of Pediatrics (AAP), and the American Academy of Family Physicians (AAFP) recommend that, in order to minimize the number of injections children receive, licensed combination vaccines may be used whenever any components of the combination are indicated and other components of the vaccine are not contraindicated *(4, 7, 13)*. Since immunization providers might not have vaccines available that contain only those antigens indicated by a child's immunization history, it is not necessary to stock all available types or brand-name products; rather, sufficient types of combination and monovalent vaccines needed to vaccinate children against all diseases for which vaccines are recommended should be stocked. Alternatively, the indicated vaccines might be available, but the provider nevertheless might prefer to use a combination vaccine to reduce the required number of injections. When patients have already received the recommended vaccinations for some of the components in a combination vaccine, administering the extra antigen(s) in the combination is often permissible if doing so will reduce the number of injections required *(4, 9)*.

In general, since the safety, immunogenicity, and efficacy of unlicensed combinations are unknown, products that are not specifically approved for mixing should not be mixed in the same syringe.

INTERCHANGEABILITY

In the case of the immunization series for an individual patient, certain vaccines from different manufacturers that protect against the same disease may be administered interchangeably in sequential doses (e.g. HepB and Hib). Combination products with similar component antigens produced by the same manufacturer (such as DTaP, DTaP-Hib, or other DTaP-combination vaccines that contain similar acellular pertussis antigens from the same manufacturer) may be used interchangeably *(9)*.

WHICH COMBINATION VACCINES ARE APPROPRIATE FOR WHICH COUNTRY? EPIDEMIOLOGIC AND ECONOMIC CONSIDERATIONS

ACIP, AAP, and AAFP recommendations on combination vaccines for childhood immunization extend beyond the United States borders. These recommendations exert a strong influence in the private practice of pediatricians, family practitioners, and other physicians who attend children around the world.

In most developing countries, immunization is carried out as a national-level program under the responsibility of the Ministry of Health. Immunization policy is driven largely by the burden of disease to be prevented by the combination vaccine in question, the public health resources available, and WHO recommendations. In the Americas, PAHO's Technical Advisory Group (TAG) on vaccine-preventable diseases has played and continues to play a pivotal, proactive role. Thus, while specific combination vaccines such as IPV and DTaP, PNV, and trivalent influenza vaccines are now the standard of care for children in the United States, OPV and DTwP are still recommended by both WHO and PAHO. In the case of the heptavalent conjugated PNV, which is a well accepted priority in most countries, both cost and supply issues have precluded its introduction into developing countries thus far. Acellular pertussis vaccines are generally better tolerated than whole-cell products. However, the difference between the two products is predominantly in the rate of mild adverse events, which do not have an impact on health as severe as that from whooping

---

BOX 1. Selected combination vaccines, and their components,
in use among children in the Americas.

Vaccine	Components
DTwP-IPV	diphtheria/tetanus/whole-cell pertussis/inactivated poliovirus vaccines
DTwP-IPV-Hib	diphtheria/tetanus/whole-cell pertussis/inactivated poliovirus/*H. influenzae* type b
DTap-IPV	diphtheria/tetanus/acellular pertussis/inactivated poliovirus vaccines
DtaP-IPV-Hib	diphtheria/tetanus/acellular pertussis/inactivated poliovirus/*H. influenzae* type b
DtwP-HBV	diphtheria/tetanus/acellular pertussis/ hepatitis B virus
DtaP	diphtheria/tetanus/acellular pertussis
MMR-V	measles/mumps/rubella/varicella
HBV-HAV	hepatitis B virus/hepatitis A virus
HBV-Hib	hepatitis B virus/*H. influenzae* type b
DTwP-HBV-Hib	diphtheria/tetanus/whole-cell pertussis/hepatitis B virus/*H. influenzae* type b
Influenza	A (H1N1), type A (H3N2), and type b

---

cough or Hib infection, both of which can be life threatening. Because of these factors, the tetravalent DTwP-Hib and the pentavalent DTwP-HepB-Hib combinations continue to be recommended by PAHO's Technical Advisory Group on vaccine-preventable diseases as the preferred vaccine for the primary series at 2, 3, and 4 months *(9)*. This recommendation is also supported by the recent experience in the United Kingdom *(30)* (see Box 1).

Many, but not all, of the new combination vaccines have been found to be safe and protective in clinical trials in developing countries under controlled conditions; however, evidence from post-marketing surveillance is often needed in order to evaluate whether the vaccine will perform equally well under field conditions once introduced into a program and sustainability can be assured *(39, 40)*.

There are other circumstances in which the introduction of a combination vaccine into the routine schedule poses dilemmas. This is the case with combination vaccines that contain Hep B vaccine as a component, which are being introduced in countries with high seroprevalence of antibodies against hepatitis B core antigen (anti-HBC). Some experts have concerns about what to do about the birth dose (the birth dose is the standard of care in the United States, as recommended by ACIP, AAP, and AAFP (4)). Since most other countries in the Region are using combination vaccines containing Hep B vaccine, a routine birth dose not only adds to the direct costs because of the need for single-dose vials, but also makes it programmatically difficult to introduce in countries with significant rural populations or marginalized urban populations. Both WHO and PAHO have established priorities for hepatitis B immunization strategies in order of importance: routine infant vaccination; prevention of perinatal HBV transmission from mother to offspring; and catch-up vaccination for older age groups. Hepatitis B seroprevalence was investigated in over 12,000 subjects in six Latin American countries or regions of countries: Argentina, Brazil's Amazon region, Chile, the Dominican Republic, Mexico, and Venezuela. Each study population was stratified according to age, gender, and socioeconomic status. Antibodies against hepatitis B core antigen (anti-HBc) were measured in order to determine hepatitis B infection. The highest overall seroprevalence was found in the Dominican Republic (21.4%), followed by Brazil (7.9%), Venezuela (3.2%), Argentina (2.1%), Mexico (1.4%), and Chile (0.6%). In all the countries, an increase in seroprevalence was found among persons aged 16 years and older, suggesting sexual transmission as the major route of infection. In addition, comparatively high seroprevalence levels were seen at an early age in the Dominican Republic and Brazil, implicating a vertical route of transmission (41).

Thus, with the exception of the Dominican Republic and Brazil's Amazon region, it usually has proved to be easiest when the three doses of hepatitis B vaccine are incorporated into the routine childhood vaccination schedule and given at the same time as the three doses of DTP, at 2, 4, and 6 months, respectively (9, 41). This schedule does not prevent perinatal hepatitis B virus infections, because it does not include a dose of hepatitis B vaccine at birth; however, this schedule does prevent infections acquired during early childhood, which account for most of the disease burden related to hepatitis B virus in countries of high disease endemicity. Over several years, as the child population gradually becomes protected against HBV infections acquired later in life, the prevalence of chronic HBV infection will decline. This process can be further accelerated by initiating an adolescent immunization campaign with a two-dose schedule where there is a documented increase in seroprevalence due to sexual transmission.

LESSONS FROM THE AMERICAS

In addition to the advantages of reducing the number of injections, combination vaccines have contributed significantly towards the harmoniza-

FIGURE 1. Annual reported rubella cases, Region of the Americas, 1982–2005.[a]

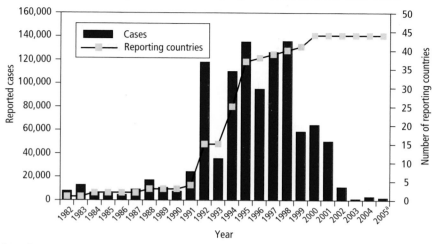

Year

[a] Data for 2005 up to week 41.

Source: Pan American Health Organization/Ministries of Health.

tion of immunization schedules of countries in the Americas. In 1992, WHO proposed including hepatitis B (HB) vaccine in countries where hepatitis B was endemic (carrier rates of 8% or greater) by 1995 and in all countries irrespective of prevalence by 1997. In 1991, the United States Advisory Committee on Immunization Practices (ACIP) recommended that both HB and Hib be included (as separate injections) into the routine universal immunization schedule for infants in that country. In 1996, WHO recommended that countries consider the use of combined DTP-HB vaccine when it became commercially available. In 1997, PAHO's Directing Council urged its Member States to strengthen surveillance in preparation for the introduction of new vaccines (such as *Haemophilus influenzae* type b, hepatitis B, and measles-mumps-rubella) to accurately determine disease burden and develop an appropriate vaccination strategy. In 1998, several countries in the Region introduced MMR to supplant the measles vaccine, thus increasing the number of vaccines in the Expanded Program on Immunization (EPI) from six to eight vaccines without changing the immunization schedule. By 2002, more than 90% of the Region's children were receiving MMR, and the countries of the Americas were documenting a significant drop in the number of registered cases of congenital rubella syndrome (CRS) (Figure 1) *(8)*.

Although *Haemophilus influenzae* type b conjugate vaccine has been available and in use in the United States and Canada since 1987, it wasn't until 1994 that Uruguay, which had a meningitis surveillance program in place, decided to include Hib vaccine in its regular immunization program. Two years later, based on a robust surveillance system and the ex-

FIGURE 2. Impact of Hib vaccination in Chile and Uruguay, up to September 1997.

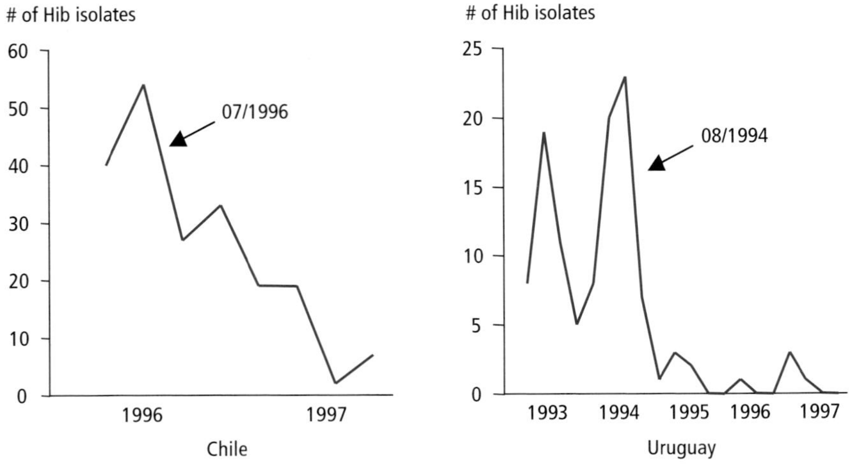

Source: Immunization Unit, Pan American Health Organization.

perience of several Hib vaccine clinical trials in the country, Chile followed suit. The impact of Hib vaccine on invasive disease in both countries was impressive (Figure 2). As the figure shows, within one year of its introduction, the incidence of invasive disease due to *Haemophilus influenzae* type b in both countries plummeted *(10)*.

By 1996, the U.S., Canada, Uruguay, and Chile were applying Hib vaccine, benefiting 4.5 million infants, representing 30% of all newborns in the Americas Region but only 3.4% of all newborns in Latin America. In 1999, with the availability of a new vaccine formulation (DTP-HepB-Hib), Mexico and Brazil joined the PAHO Revolving Fund and, due to large-volume purchases helped reduce the price of Hib—the price of the vaccine had ranged from US$ 4.00 to US$ 8.50 when purchased directly from the manufacturers, and dropped to a record low of $3.50 (including DTwP and Hep B). By participating in the revolving fund, these two countries were able to introduce both Hib and Hep B without changing their immunization schedules. The lowered prices had an important impact on the prices of the monovalent Hib and DTP-Hib due to competition, which allowed other countries in the Region to incorporate Hib into their regular immunization program. By 2000, it was estimated that 15,889,000 infants, 92% of all newborns in the Region and 89% of all newborns in Latin America, had received Hib and hepatitis B vaccines (Figure 3). Since then, many countries in the Americas have introduced combination vaccines that contain Hib, Hep B, or both, such as in the DTwP-HB-Hib pentavalent vaccine *(10)*.

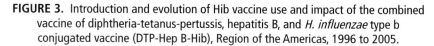

FIGURE 3. Introduction and evolution of Hib vaccine use and impact of the combined vaccine of diphtheria-tetanus-pertussis, hepatitis B, and *H. influenzae* type b conjugated vaccine (DTP-Hep B-Hib), Region of the Americas, 1996 to 2005.

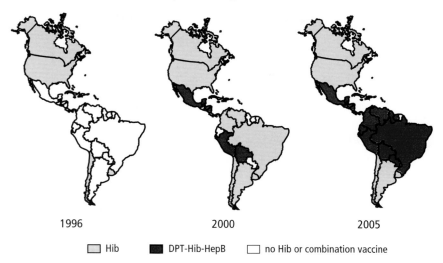

| 1996 | 2000 | 2005 |

☐ Hib   ■ DPT-Hib-HepB   ☐ no Hib or combination vaccine

Source: Country reports to the Pan American Health Organization.

COST ISSUES

One of the leading deterrents for introducing new vaccines has been their price. New combination vaccines are expected to cost more than traditional childhood vaccines. Thus, before introducing a new combination vaccine, or any vaccine for that matter, it is important to conduct economic evaluations looking at the actual vaccine and operating costs in the context of the country's public health expenditure. Equally important is being able to guarantee the sustainability of the vaccine in the program once introduced, which often is determined more by guaranteed supply than cost issues (11, 42).

The introduction of combination vaccines in Mexico between 1956 and 2004 (Box 2) has had remarkable effects, as evidenced by recent developments. When Mexico adopted WHO's EPI, the immunization schedule consisted of six vaccines—two combination vaccines, IPV (which was later supplanted by OPV), BCG, DTP, and measles. The schedule remained unchanged for 25 years until 1998, when MMR supplanted the measles monovalent vaccine. Successful field trials with DTP-HepB-Hib carried out in Mexico and other countries in the Region permitted this combination vaccine to be introduced in place of DTwP in 1999 (21). Combination vaccines also have been introduced into the adolescent immu-

BOX 2. Introduction of combination vaccines,
Mexico, 1956–2004.

Year	Vaccine
1956	Introduction of Salk's trivalent IPV
1961	Diphtheria, tetanus, pertussis (2, 4, 6 mos.)
1962	IPV supplanted by Sabin's OPV
1973	Introduction of the Universal EPI Program (BCG, OPV, DTP, and measles)
1997	TT substituted by Td as booster (12 yrs.)
1998	MMR (12 mos., booster at 6 yrs.)
1998	DTwP-hepatitis B, *H. influenzae* type b (2, 4, 6 mos.)
2000	Td, MR, & HB for adolescents (12–19 yrs.)
2004	Trivalent influenza (6–23 mos.)

nization schedule: the tetanus booster was supplanted by Td, and MR was added to the adolescent schedule in an effort to eliminate neonatal tetanus, protect against diphtheria, and accelerate the containment of wild measles and the elimination of congenital rubella syndrome. Concerned about the impending influenza pandemic, Mexico's National Immunization Council (CONAVA) introduced the trivalent influenza vaccine in 2004 as part of the national immunization program for infants between 6 and 23 months *(43)*.

Over an eight-year period (1997–2004), with the introduction of combination vaccines, Mexico's immunization schedule almost doubled, increasing from six to 11 vaccines. Because combination vaccines were incorporated into the existing schedule, the number of injections did not change. During the same period, the vaccine cost increased significantly, from a low of US$ 1.40 for the complete EPI schedule to US$ 13.50 when measles was supplanted by MMR and DTwP by DTP-HepB-Hib. The reasons behind the success of Hib vaccine introduction in the Region can be attributed to the existence of strong EPI programs in the countries together with strong leadership at PAHO's central and country levels *(44)*.

REMAINING CHALLENGES

The future of combination vaccines in the 21st century will play an important role in future childhood immunization strategies. Combination vaccines present unique challenges and opportunities for manufacturing and product development. Vaccine development should focus on generating strong, broad-based immunity to several antigens from a number of pathogens using combination methodologies to the extent possible. The advances in molecular biology and genetic engineering will play an important role in developing new combination vaccines, including DNA vaccines and conjugate vaccines. Alternative means of multiple antigen delivery by the mucosal and cutaneous routes are also being explored *(45)*.

Achieving optimal safety and effectiveness for all vaccines is a top priority, particularly because vaccines are administered to healthy children. The pre-licensing evaluation of combination vaccines composed of previously licensed components or of novel antigens will require well-designed and well-coordinated multinational prospective clinical trials with realistic sample sizes and appropriate control groups. The major task ahead for anticipating the introduction of existing or new combination vaccines requires the joint participation of several government ministries, investigators, private and public vaccine manufacturers, international and local regulatory agencies, international agencies, and the public at large. The success of these public health strategies will depend on the extent to which countries place a value on the benefit of vaccines, and accordingly make vaccines available to their populations and guarantee their sustainability once introduced. It is important to underscore that there is a difference between vaccines being cheap and being affordable *(11, 45, 46)*. Lessons learned from the Americas demonstrate that through political will, combined with innovative financing and consolidated purchasing strategies, new combination vaccines can be introduced and used in immunization programs by countries, regardless of their income level.

References

1. Centers for Disease Control and Prevention. Ten great public health achievements: United States, 1900–1999. *MMWR* 1999;48(12):241–243.
2. Postema AS, Myers MG, Breiman RF. Challenges in the development, licensure, and use of combination vaccines. *Clin Infect Dis* 2001;33(4 suppl): S261–S266.
3. Centers for Disease Control and Prevention. Notice to readers: recommended childhood immunization schedule—United States, 2000. *MMWR* 2000;49(47): 35–38.
4. Centers for Disease Control and Prevention. Notice to readers: recommended childhood immunization scheduleUnited States, 2005. *MMWR* 2005;53(51): Q1–Q3.
5. Woodin KA, Rodewald LE, Humiston SG, Carges MS, Schaffer SJ, Szilagyi PG. Physician and parent opinions. Are children becoming pincushions from immunizations? *Arch Pediatr Adolesc Med* 1995;149(8):845–849.
6. Vivier PM, Alario AJ, Peter G, Leddy T, Simon P, Mor V. An analysis of the immunization status of preschool children enrolled in a statewide Medicaid managed care program. *J Pediatr* 2001;139(5):624–629.

7. Centers for Disease Control and Prevention. National, state, and urban area vaccination coverage levels among children aged 19–35 months—United States, 1997. *MMWR* 1997;47(26):547–554.

8. Dietz V, Venczel L, Izurieta H, et al. Assessing and monitoring vaccination coverage levels: lessons from the Americas. *Rev Panam Salud Publica* 2004; 16(6):432–442.

9. Decker MD, Edwards KM, Bogaerts HH. Combination vaccines. In: Plotkin SA, Orenstein WA, eds. *Vaccines*. 4th ed. Philadelphia: WB Saunders, 2004;825–861.

10. Di Fabio JL and de Quadros, C. Considerations for combination vaccine development. *Clin Infect Dis* 2001;33(4 suppl):S340–S345.

11. Weniger BG, Chen RT, Jacobson SH. Addressing the challenges to immunization practice with an economic algorithm for vaccine selection. *Vaccine* 1998;16 (19):1885–1897.

12. Dietz VJ, Stevenson J, Zell ER, Cochi S, Hadler S, Eddins D. Potential impact on vaccination coverage levels by administering vaccines simultaneously and reducing dropout rates. *Arch Pediatr Adolesc Med* 1994;148(9):943–949.

13. American Academy of Pediatrics. Combination Vaccines for Childhood Immunization: Recommendations of the Advisory Committee on Immunization Practices (ACIP), the American Academy of Pediatrics (AAP), and the American Academy of Family Physicians (AAFP). *Pediatrics* 1999;103(5 Pt 1):1064–1077.

14. Usonis V, Bakasenas V, Willems P, Clemens R. Feasibility study of a combined diphtheria-tetanus-acellular pertussis-hepatitis B (DTPa-HBV) vaccine and comparison of clinical responses with diphtheria tetanus-acellular pertussis (DTaP) and hepatitis B vaccines applied as mixed or injected separate limbs. *Vaccine* 1997;15(15):1680–1686.

15. Dagan R, Igbaria K, Piglansky L, et al. Safety and immunogenicity of a combined pentavalent diphtheria, tetanus, acellular pertussis inactivated poliovirus and *Haemophilus influenzae* type b-tetanus conjugate vaccine in infants, compared with a whole cell pertussis pentavalent vaccine. *Pediatr Infect Dis J* 1997;16(12):1113–1121.

16. Halsey NA. Safety of combination vaccines: perception versus reality. *Pediatr Infect Dis J* 2001;20(11 suppl):S40–S44.

17. Yeh SH, et al. Safety and immunogenicity of a pentavalent diphtheria, tetanus, pertussis, hepatitis B and polio combination vaccine in infants. *Pediatr Infect Dis J* 2001;20(10):973–980.

18. Elliman D, Bedford H. Safety and efficacy of combination vaccines. *BMJ* 2003; 326(7397):995–996.

19. Taffs RE. Potency tests of combination vaccines. *Clin Infect Dis* 2001;33 (4 suppl): S362–S366.

20. Faingezicht I, Avila-Aguerro ML, Cervantes Y, Fourneau M, Costa Clemens SA. Primary and booster vaccination with DTPw-HB/Hib pentavalent vaccine in Costa Rican children who had received a birth dose of hepatitis B vaccine. *Rev Panam Salud Publica* 2002;12(4):247–257.

21. Santos JI, Martin A, De Leon T, Rivera L, Gaitan ME, Del Rio C, Oselka G, Cervantes Y, Rubio P, Clemens SA, de Mendonca JS. DTPw-HB and Hib primary and booster vaccination: combined versus separate administration to Latin American children. *Vaccine* 2002;20(13–14):1887–1893.

22. Granoff DM, Rappuoli R. Are serological responses to acellular pertussis antigens sufficient criteria to ensure that new combination vaccines are effective for prevention of disease? *Dev Biol Stand* 1997;89:379–389.
23. Tiru M, Hallander HO, Gustafsson L, Storsaeter J, Olin P. Diphtheria antitoxin response to DTP vaccines used in Swedish pertussis vaccine trials, persistence and projection for timing of booster. *Vaccine* 2000;18(21):2295–2306.
24. Pichichero ME, Latiolais T, Bernstein DI, Hosbach P, Christian E, Vidor E, et al. Vaccine antigen interactions after a combination diphtheria-tetanus toxoid-acellular pertussis/purified capsular polysaccharide of *Haemophilus influenzae* type b-tetanus toxoid vaccine in two-, four- and six-month-old infants. *Pediatr Infect Dis J* 1997;16:863–870.
25. Lee CY, Thipphawong J, Huang LM, et al. An evaluation of the safety and immunogenicity of a five-component acellular pertussis, diphtheria, and tetanus toxoid vaccine (DTaP) when combined with a *Haemophilus influenzae* type b-tetanus toxoid conjugate vaccine (PRP-T) in Taiwanese infants. *Pediatrics* 1999;103(1):25–30.
26. Eskola J, Ward J, Dagan R, Goldblatt D, Zepp F, Siegrist CA. Combined vaccination of *Haemophilus influenzae* type b conjugate and diphtheria-tetanus-pertussis containing acellular pertussis. *Lancet* 1999;354(9195):2063–2068.
27. Daum RS, Zenko CE, Given GZ, Ballanco GA, Parikh H, Germino K. Magnitude of interference after diphtheria-tetanus toxoids-acellular pertussis/*Haemophilus influenzae* type b capsular polysaccharide-tetanus vaccination is related to the number of doses administered. *J Infect Dis* 2001;184(10):1293–1299.
28. Vidor E, Hoffenbach A, Fletcher MA. *Haemophilus influenzae* type b vaccine: reconstitution of lyophilized PRP-T vaccine with a pertussis-containing pediatric combination vaccine, or a change in the primary series immunization schedule, may modify the serum anti-PRP antibody responses. *Curr Med Res Opin* 2001;17(3):197–209.
29. Trotter CL, Ramsay ME, Slack MPE. Rising incidence of *Haemophilus influenzae* type b disease in England and Wales indicates a need for a second catch-up vaccination campaign. *Commun Dis Public Health* 2003;6(1):55–58.
30. Johnson NG, Ruggeberg JU, Balfour GF, Chen Lee Y, Liddy H, Irving D, Sheldon, J, et al. *Haemophilus influenzae* type b reemergence after combination immunization. *Emerg Infect Dis* 2006;12(6):937–939.
31. Dagan R, Eskola J, Leclerc C, Leroy O. Reduced response to multiple vaccines sharing common protein epitopes that are administered simultaneously to infants. *Infect Immun* 1998;66(5):2093–2098.
32. Buttery JP, Riddell A, McVernon J, Chantler T, Lane L, Bowen-Morris J, Diggle L, et al. Immunogenicity and safety of a combination pneumococcal-meningococcal vaccine in infants. *JAMA* 2005;293(14):1751–1758.
33. Halsey NA. Combination vaccines: defining and addressing current safety concerns. *Clin Infect Dis* 2001;33(4 suppl):S312–S318.
34. Schmitt HJ, Knuf M, Ortiz E, Sänger R, Uwamwezi MC, Kaufbold A. Primary vaccination of infants with diphtheria-tetanus-acellular pertussis-hepatitis B virus-inactivated polio virus and *Haemophilus influenzae* type b vaccines given as either separate or mixed injections. *J Pediatr* 2000;137(3):304–312.

35. Wakefield AJ, Murch SH, Anthony A, Linnell J, Casson DM, Malik M, et al. Ileal-lymphoid nodular hyperplasia, non-specific colitis, and pervasive developmental disorder in children. *Lancet* 1998;351(9103):637–641.
36. Miller E. MMR vaccine: review of benefits and risks. *J Infect* 2002;44(1):1–6.
37. Offit PA, Quarles J, Gerber MA, Hackett CJ, Marcuse EK, Kollman TR, et al. Addressing parents' concerns: do multiple vaccines overwhelm or weaken the infant's immune system? *Pediatrics* 2002;109(1):124–129.
38. Pichichero ME, Cernichiari E, Lopreiato J, Treanor J. Mercury concentrations and metabolism in infants receiving vaccines containing thiomersal: a descriptive study. *Lancet* 2002;360(9347):1737–1741.
39. Clemens J, Brenner R, Rao M, Tafari N, Lowe C. Evaluating new vaccines for developing countries. Efficacy or effectiveness? *JAMA* 1996;275(5):390–397.
40. Clemens J, Jodar L. Introducing new vaccines into developing countries: obstacles, opportunities and complexities. *Nature Med* 2005;11(4 suppl): S12–S15.
41. Silveira TR, da Fonseca JC, Rivera L, Fay OH, Tapia R, Santos JI, Urdeneta E, Clemens SAC. Hepatitis B seroprevalence in Latin America. *Rev Panam Salud Publica* 1999;6(6):378–383.
42. Mahoney R. Policy analysis: an essential research tool for the introduction of vaccines in developing countries. *J Health Popul Nutr* 2004;22(3):331–337.
43. Santos JI. Cambio estratégico en el programa de vacunación universal de México: vacunación contra influenza en población pediátrica de 23–26 meses. *Bol Med Hosp Inf Mex* 2004;61:461–464.
44. Frenk-Mora J, Tapia-Conyer R, and Santos JI. A vision for the national financing of immunization programs. In: de Quadros C, ed. *Vaccines: preventing disease and protecting health.* Washington, DC: Pan American Health Organization, 2003:333–340.
45. Hinman AR. Perspectives on the state of combination vaccines: summary of the rapporteur for the International Symposium on Combination Vaccines. *Clin Infect Dis* 2001 Dec 15;33(4 suppl):S372–S375.
46. Andrus JK, Tambini G, Di Fabio JL, et al. Anticipating new vaccines in the Americas. *Rev Panam Salud Publica* 2004;16(6):369–370.

OPTIMAL USE OF BCG VACCINE

Mauricio L. Barreto, MD, MPH, PhD,[1]
Susan M. Pereira, MD, MPH,[1] *and Sergio S. Cunha, MD, MPH*[1]

INTRODUCTION

Tuberculosis is a major public health problem today, with more than 50 million people infected with the tubercle bacillus (*Mycobacterium tuberculosis*). It is estimated that more than six million new cases and two million deaths occur each year. Latent tuberculosis infection (LTBI) is estimated to be present in more than two billion people worldwide. Due to certain known factors (such as any condition inducing immunological deficiency), a small proportion of the total LTBI cases develop into clinical TB cases. The most frequent manifestation of TB is pulmonary TB, which is also the form that most contributes to the dissemination of *M. tuberculosis* and, as a consequence, deserves great public health attention. In developing countries, the incidence of TB has remained consistently high over the past few decades. In those countries with a high AIDS burden, this incidence has increased sharply (1). In industrialized countries, the increase in the incidence of TB was associated with an increase in the incidence of AIDS and, in some locations, with increased poverty or social inequalities (2).

In countries with a low prevalence of TB, control programs emphasize the identification and treatment of individuals with LTBI, in order to prevent them from becoming new clinical cases, as well as the early identification and treatment of cases. One of the principal arguments used in favor of the discontinuation of BCG vaccination in some of these countries has been the fact that BCG interferes with the result of the tuberculin skin test (TST), the traditional way of diagnosing LTBI. In developing countries with a high TB burden, however, TB control measures include neona-

[1] Institute of Collective Health, Federal University of Bahia, Bahia, Brazil.

tal BCG vaccination, as well as diagnosis and treatment of TB cases and chemoprophylaxis among contacts of TB cases (3).

BCG vaccine has been used worldwide and is produced by different manufacturers around the world. BCG is derived from an attenuated species of virulent bovine tubercle bacillus developed by Calmette and Guérin. In 1908, these two investigators began to develop a series of sub-cultures of a virulent *M. bovis* bacillus by applying 231 culture cycles with transfers every three weeks on a glycerol-potato-bile medium. After 13 years, an attenuated strain of *M. bovis* was obtained, referred to as the "bacillus of Calmette-Guérin (BCG)." The vaccine derived from this bacillus became the first human TB vaccine, and remains the only one to this day (4).

BCG vaccines produced by different manufacturers are similar, though not identical, in several of their bacteriological characteristics. These differences occur due to the biological variability within different strains, which are genotypically and phenotypically distinct. Therefore, the characteristics of the BCG vaccine differ with respect to certain aspects of viability, immunogenicity, reactogenicity, and residual virulence, depending on the strain used by the manufacturer. More recent genomic studies have demonstrated that different BCG strains also differ in some genetic characteristics (5).

The vaccine, used for the first time in 1921, was administered orally to the newborn infant of a mother infected with tuberculosis; the child showed no adverse effects. Although BCG vaccine has some side effects, it is generally considered safe. An unfortunate adverse event related to the administration of BCG vaccine occurred in 1929–1930 in Lübeck, Germany. An oral BCG vaccine contaminated with virulent tubercle bacilli was administered to children. Of the 251 infants vaccinated, 73 died (6).

In 1927, intradermal administration of the BCG vaccine was introduced. As part of the effort to combat TB, BCG was largely adopted in Europe over the following years. By 1939, a multiple puncture vaccination method was developed (3, 4, 7). Beginning in 1930, the first clinical trials to evaluate first-dose protection were initiated. Based on study results that showed BCG to be very effective, the World Health Organization (WHO) and the United Nations Children's Fund (UNICEF) began recommending BCG vaccination campaigns around the world. WHO has been recommending that the first BCG-vaccine dose be given since 1948 (3). It is estimated that 1.5 billion people received the BCG vaccine between 1948 and 1974. In 1974, the BCG vaccine was incorporated into the infant vaccination schedule of the Expanded Program on Immunization (EPI). Today, BCG vaccination is recommended in practically every country in the world, and it is estimated that approximately 100 million children receive the vaccine each year. Worldwide, BCG vaccination coverage at the end of the 1990s reached 85% of all newborn infants. The lowest vaccination levels have been registered in Africa, Southeast Asia, and the Western Pacific regions (3).

Originally developed for the prevention of tuberculosis, the BCG vaccine has recently been shown to have a protective effect against other mycobacterioses, particularly leprosy and Buruli ulcer (8). It also has been effective in immunotherapy of some forms of cancer, especially bladder cancer (9). Unproven isolated findings have been reported, including protective effects against hookworm (10) and other helminth infections (11). There also have been reports in the literature of a reduced incidence of atopy in children vaccinated with BCG (12, 13).

CONTROVERSIES ABOUT THE EFFECT OF BCG'S FIRST DOSE ON PULMONARY TUBERCULOSIS

Several studies have been conducted to evaluate the protective efficacy of BCG against TB. Depending on aspects of study design or on the geographic areas where the study was conducted, huge variations have been found in the efficacy level. These variations in protective efficacy have raised concerns regarding some of the vaccine's uses. Interestingly, these concerns have become more controversial as new information has emerged in recent decades. For instance, today there is considerable consensus about the degree of protection that the first BCG dose offers against severe forms of tuberculosis in children (principally meningitis and miliary disease); however, experts continue to debate the protective effect of BCG on pulmonary TB, which is the main target of TB control.

As has been expressed since the 1930s, several clinical trials have been conducted to evaluate the efficacy of the first BCG dose against TB. Regarding pulmonary TB, results have shown a range of efficacy that varies between 0% and 80% (14–20). The last trial, which was also the largest one, was performed in Madras, India, and showed no protection whatsoever. This serves to highlight the complexity of the current BCG debate. Variation in these findings has served to increase the degree of uncertainty among the TB control community concerning the protective effect of the BCG vaccine against pulmonary TB (7, 21).

The case-control studies, performed to evaluate the effectiveness of the first BCG dose in protecting against TB, reported protective efficacies that ranged from 6% to 73% for all forms of TB. Of note is the outcome measure in the majority of case-control studies in pulmonary TB cases. Specific protection against pulmonary tuberculosis varied between 10% and 66%. For meningeal and miliary TB less variability was found and the minimum protection reported was above 50%. Certainly, these studies differ from each other in several aspects of study design, including age of the cases or the study population, clinical forms and diagnosis of TB, control selection, and sample size (22–37). Other case-control studies conducted among HIV-infected children have shown no evidence of BCG protection against pulmonary or extra-pulmonary forms of TB (38, 39).

Data from several randomized controlled trials and case-control studies have been used in several meta-analyses, producing summarized estimates of the effect of the BCG vaccine. The protection against tuberculous meningitis and miliary TB was homogenous and high in all the meta-analysis studies, producing a pooled estimate of protective effect of 86% (40). Pooled protective effect for all forms of TB was similar to the results from the randomized control trials and case-control studies, 51% and 50%, respectively (41). The results of the pooled estimates of the effect of the BCG vaccine against pulmonary tuberculosis should be viewed with caution. Because of the very high degree of heterogeneity among the studies used, some experts considered the meta-analyses inappropriate for making summarized estimations of the vaccine's protective effect (42).

WHY IS THE EFFECT OF BCG ON PULMONARY TUBERCULOSIS SO VARIABLE?

The variation in BCG protection has been attributed to the following four factors:

- **Biological variability in BCG due to different strains.** This effect is due to BCG strain mutations and immunogenic differences between strains cultured in different laboratories over many years. Different studies conducted in different countries with the same BCG strain had discordant results with respect to efficacy estimates (21, 43, 44).
- **Exposure to environmental mycobacteria.** Environmental mycobacteria (EM) may result in interactions with the receptor immune system, interfering with BCG protection. Clinical trials performed in countries lying far from the equator, which are characterized by a low prevalence of environmental mycobacteria, reported higher efficacy estimates. The low efficacy estimates reported in southern India are concordant with acquired heterologous immunity through exposure to environmental mycobacteria. Meta-analysis studies suggest that 41% of the variation in efficacy estimates may be explained by the latitude variation, as a proxy of environmental-mycobacteria exposure (21, 44, 45).
- **Route of infection.** BCG has been shown to be highly protective when tuberculosis is caused by the mechanism of primary infection (tuberculosis meningitis, for example) and to offer reduced protection when tu-

berculosis is caused by exogenous reinfection. If this hypothesis is true, BCG would offer lower protection in high-infection risk populations with a high occurrence of exogenous reinfection (20).

• **Factors related to vaccine administration.** Many factors are related to BCG use, such as viability, dose, route of administration, inappropriate storage or transportation of the vaccine, and vaccination technique. Host factors such as nutritional status, occurrence of concurrent infections, and genetic characteristics also play a role (20, 46, 47).

To summarize, while evidence supports the EM hypothesis, it still remains a hypothesis with no definitive proof.

DURATION OF THE BCG EFFECT

Knowing how long neonatal BCG protection lasts is critical for taking rational policy decisions on vaccination (1). Evidence so far suggests that BCG protection wanes over time (48), and until recently there was no evidence that protection against pulmonary disease lasted for more than 15 years following vaccination. However, a recent paper has reported protection lasting over six decades in American Indians and Alaskan natives who participated in a placebo-controlled BCG vaccine trial started in 1935–1938 and who were still at risk for developing tuberculosis (49). Another study using the control arm of a trial on the efficacy of revaccination in schoolchildren in Brazil showed substantial protection of neonatal BCG vaccination lasting 15–20 years against all forms of tuberculosis (50). If confirmed, these two recently published studies suggest that BCG protection may last much longer than previously believed.

BCG REVACCINATION

Given that the protective effect of the BCG vaccination wanes over time and that a booster dose may be able to increase the effect of the vaccine, repeated doses of BCG have been routinely used in some countries, such as Chile, Hungary, Portugal, and Russia. However, WHO's global programs on tuberculosis and on vaccines do not recommend repeated BCG vaccination, since there is no conclusive evidence to determine whether or not it confers added protection (51). Indeed, a great part of the evidence in favor or against BCG revaccination comes from inconclusive observational studies. In Hungary, BCG revaccination has been used since 1959 in the population under 20 years of age with no tuberculin response to purified protein derivative (PPD). Rapid decrease in the incidence of TB was observed in revaccinated children when compared with the non-revaccinated adult population, and this has been explained as being an effect of BCG revaccination (52). A case-control study performed in Chile, where BCG revaccination has been adopted, failed to find any protective effect (53). In Finland, the second BCG dose was discontinued after 1990 because no increase in protective effect was observed against the incidence of tuberculosis (54). The only published randomized control trial results that aimed to evaluate the effect of BCG revaccination was conducted in the general population of Malawi; results showed no protection against TB, but did show a 50% reduction in cases of leprosy (55). Of note, the first dose was not protective against TB in this country either. In Brazil, results of a large randomized control trial conducted among schoolchildren in two cities found no BCG revaccination protection against tuberculosis (56) or leprosy. Leprosy results have not yet been published (57).

BCG SCAR

BCG vaccination usually leaves a scar at the injection site (58). The BCG scar is considered a good indicator of previous BCG vaccination. In two cities in Brazil, the sensitivity and specificity of BCG scar reading was very high for previous vaccination (59, 60). However, it has been demonstrated by other authors that 17% to 25% of BCG-vaccinated children have no scar (61, 62). There is no conclusive evidence of any association between the presence of a BCG scar and vaccine protection. Scar size is affected by tuberculin response prior to vaccination. It was observed that individuals with a greater pre-vaccination tuberculin response had scars 2.8 mm larger (63). Small BCG scars have been described when a lower BCG dose was administered (0.05 ml) (64). A positive association between BCG scar size and the number of vaccinations is documented in the literature (62, 65).

TUBERCULIN SKIN TEST RESPONSE AND BCG VACCINATION

Tuberculin skin test (TST) response measures the degree of allergy to the tuberculin protein. BCG vaccination interferes with the TST response, principally when the skin test is performed within 15 years of BCG vaccination. TST responses obtained when BCG was given after infancy were higher (RR 10, 95% CI 5.29 to 18.89) than following neonatal BCG (RR 2.4, 95% CI 2.00 to 2.97). A post-vaccination reaction to a tuberculin test is no longer considered an indicator of BCG vaccine-induced immunity (66, 67). There is no evidence that delayed-type reactions following BCG vaccination are associated with vaccine protection.

BCG AND LEPROSY

BCG was originally developed to prevent tuberculosis, but soon the hypothesis was raised regarding whether BCG vaccination could also prevent leprosy. Since the 1960s, several studies have been conducted. Seven controlled trials were carried out in six countries (7, 68). For the general population, vaccine protection varied from having no effect whatsoever (in Brazil) (69) to 50% efficacy (in Malawi) (7); these were estimates from studies evaluating the second dose. For the first dose, the vaccine protection ranged from 14% in India (in the general population) to 80% (among contacts). There were 14 case-control studies aimed at evaluating the effect of the BCG vaccine on leprosy (12 studies on first dose) (7, 70–73). In 13 of these studies, BCG had been administered to the population routinely as part of the TB control effort. In one study, the BCG vaccination was given to leprosy contacts as a routine health practice (74). Estimates of overall vaccine protection with statistically significant results were observed in 12 case-control studies and varied from 36% (75) to 90% (71). In two studies, protection was observed only in the case of specific clinical forms of the disease (76, 77). Therefore, there is consistent evidence that a first-dose BCG vaccine provides protection against leprosy. There also is some evidence that an additional dose confers additional protection (55, 74, 78). However, the estimates of this protection varied, and attempts to conduct pooled estimates were difficult to interpret. Therefore, despite the high protection found in some studies (7, 13) the impact of such a vaccination against leprosy cannot be easily generalized. Questions regarding whom, how often, and when to vaccinate for leprosy control have not yet been answered (79).

In Brazil, where for several years BCG vaccination/revaccination has been officially recommended to household contacts of leprosy cases, the real benefits of such a strategy in terms of its impact on the incidence of leprosy in the community and its cost-effectiveness have not yet been demonstrated (80).

Should, then, BCG vaccination be recommended as protection against leprosy? One of the by-products of the first dose of neonatal BCG may be its protective effect against leprosy (13). Recommending the vaccination of contacts of leprosy cases remains in question, however. Given the evidence so far, it would seem that the impact of BCG vaccination targeted specifically against leprosy among contacts is not easily predictable and should, therefore, only be recommended under strict scrutiny. Its impact will depend on the effectiveness of a second-dose vaccine among children and adults, and on the proportion of leprosy cases in the general population which originated from contacts (80). Where such strategies have already been implemented, it is advisable to conduct well-designed studies to evaluate their impact.

ADVERSE EVENTS RELATED TO BCG

The most frequent adverse events are local ulcers and regional suppura-tive lymphadenitis (SL). The incidence rates of adverse events ranged from 0.1 per 1,000 vaccinated children in Denmark to 5.0 per 1,000 vacci-nated children in some developing countries (81). Most of the SL cases occur during the first five months after vaccination. Fatal dissemination of BCG is a rare event—with an incidence rate of only 0.19 to 1.56 per 1 mil-lion vaccinees—and occurs when individuals with severely depressed cel-lular immunity are inadvertently vaccinated. Other rare events are cases of BCG osteitis, with an estimated rate of 0.6 to 46 cases per 1 million vac-cinated children (81). The development of progressive immunosuppres-sion may lead to a reactivation of latent BCG organisms, causing regional or disseminated adverse events. Disseminated adverse events have been described in AIDS patients. The number of known cases is low, probably due to underreporting because diagnosis requires the availability of labo-ratory facilities (82). The occurrence of adverse events correlates with the bacterial concentration of the vaccine, the age at vaccination, the BCG strain used in the vaccine, and the vaccination technique used. Revaccina-tion does not appear to significantly increase the frequency of adverse events associated with BCG use (83).

BCG AND HIV/AIDS

The HIV/AIDS epidemic has contributed to an increase in the incidence of tuberculosis in several countries in the developing and in the devel-oped world. The main explanation for this increase is that HIV/AIDS pa-tients frequently have severely depressed immune systems that favor the reactivation of latent tuberculosis infection (LTBI). The main concern re-garding the control of TB among HIV/AIDS patients is the role of BCG vaccination. It is known that children with immunodeficiency syndromes more frequently develop lymphadenitis or disseminated BCG disease after vaccination. WHO recommends that asymptomatic children living in countries with a high prevalence of tuberculosis be vaccinated with BCG, but that symptomatic HIV-infected children not be vaccinated. In general, countries with a low prevalence of TB tend not to adopt BCG vac-cination for individuals known to be HIV-infected (84).

BCG IN TB PREVENTION—ROUTINE USE

In a vast majority of countries, vaccination with a first dose of BCG is rou-tine practice, with countries varying only in terms of the age group to be targeted and the number of doses to be administered. Only a few countries in the world—the United States and the Netherlands among them—do not recommend routine BCG vaccination for their populations. In countries with a high burden of TB, there is no doubt that a single dose of BCG vaccine must be given to infants soon after birth. WHO recommends intradermal application in the arm's deltoid region using a syringe and needle. A few countries adopted percutaneus administration with a multiple puncture technique. The recommended dose is 0.1 ml, applied intradermically in the lower section of the right deltoid muscle. This recommendation is based on the high effectiveness of the BCG vaccine in protecting against disseminated tuberculosis in children, or other serious presentations (3). In the United Kingdom and in some other European countries, the first dose of BCG is given to school-aged children (between 12 and 13 years of age) with a negative tuberculin skin test. Repeated BCG has been used in several countries. Portugal and Switzerland recommend two doses, while Russia and other eastern European countries have adopted up to five doses. Nevertheless, as already discussed, there is no evidence to support administering more than one dose of the vaccine (7, 85).

ADMINISTERING BCG TO HEALTH-CARE WORKERS

Health-care workers have a higher incidence of tuberculosis compared to other professional categories. Recently, nosocomial outbreaks of tuberculosis have been reported, some of them caused by multidrug-resistant strains. In countries with a low prevalence of TB, nosocomial transmission has been described in clusters of patients and health-care workers (86). Many experts agree that BCG vaccination should be encouraged among unvaccinated health-care personnel with negative tuberculin skin tests (7, 84) (see Box 1).

WILL BCG BE SUBSTITUTED? STATUS OF THE DEVELOPMENT OF NEW TB VACCINES

In the developing world, the advantages of using BCG surpass the vaccine's deficiencies, which include its variable effect on pulmonary tuberculosis depending on geographic location, the difficult interpretation of the tuberculin skin test, and the fact that it is unsafe for patients with depressed immune systems. This is not the case in industrialized countries, however, and a huge effort is now under way to identify new TB vaccines. The ideal vaccine must overcome the deficiencies of the BCG vaccine and must, in particular, be effective following exposure to M. tuberculosis. In addition, vaccines to be used as adjunctive immunotherapy associated

---

BOX 1. Summary of BCG vaccination recommendations.

Who Should Be Vaccinated
- Newborns living in areas where TB prevalence is moderate to high.
- Infants and children at particular risk of TB exposure in low endemic areas.
- Asymptomatic HIV-infected children who are at high risk for infection.
- Health-care workers previously unvaccinated, TST negative or Heaf test grade 1 [corresponding to Mantoux negative, (<5 mm) performed using 10 TU (0.1ml/100 TU/m)].

Who Should Not Be Vaccinated
- Infants and children with symptomatic human immunodeficiency virus (HIV) or those known to have any other immunodeficiency condition.
- Patients under immunosuppressive treatment (corticosteroids, alkylating agents, antimetabolites, radiation).
- Pregnant women.

---

with conventional treatment have already been conceived. Hundreds of candidate vaccines using different concepts have been developed and a few are already undergoing Phase I or Phase II trials. Phase III trials are expected to start soon (87–89).

Additional concerns remain regarding the testing and introduction of new TB vaccines, specifically in countries with a high TB burden. In some countries, the remarkable impact of the BCG vaccine on miliary and meningitis TB in childhood is sufficient reason to justify its use. Consequently, there is a consensus that on scientific and ethical grounds a new TB vaccine should be tested in childhood populations previously vaccinated with BCG (90). Only when the benefits of a new vaccine have been completely clarified should replacement of the BCG vaccine be undertaken.

References

1. Grant AD, De Cock KM. The growing challenge of HIV/AIDS in developing countries. *Br Med Bull* 1998;54(2):369–381.
2. Tocque K, Doherty MJ, Bellis MA, Spence DP, Williams CS, Davies PD. Tuberculosis notifications in England: the relative effects of deprivation and immigration. *Int J Tuber Lung Dis* 1998;2(3):213–218.
3. WHO. Global tuberculosis control: surveillance, planning, financing: WHO Report 2004. Geneva, Switzerland, 2004.
4. Lugosi L. Theoretical and methodological aspects of BCG vaccine from the discovery of Calmette and Guerin to molecular biology. A review. *Tuber Lung Dis* 1992;73(5):252–261.
5. Behr MA. BCG—different strains, different vaccines? *Lancet Infect Dis* 2002; Feb 2(2):86–92.

6. CDC. The role of BCG vaccine in the prevention and control of tuberculosis. *MMWR* 1996;45(N R 44).

7. Fine PEM, Carneiro IAM, Milstien JB, Clements CJ. Issues relating to the use of BCG in immunization programmes. A discussion document. Geneva: World Health Organization, 1999:45.

8. Dai G, McMurray DN. Altered cytokine production and impaired antimyco-bacterial immunity in protein-malnourished guinea pigs. *Infect Immun* 1998; 66(8):3562–3568.

9. Sylvester RJ, van der Meidjen AP, Lamm DL. Intravesical bacillus Calmette-Guerin reduces the risk of progression in patients with superficial bladder cancer: a meta-analysis of the published results of randomized clinical trials. *J Urol* 2002;168(5):1964–1970.

10. Barreto ML, Rodrigues LC, Silva RCR, et al. Lower hookworm incidence, prevalence, and intensity of infection in children with a bacillus Calmette-Guerin vaccination scar. *J Infect Dis* 2000;182(6):1800–1803.

11. Elliott AM, Nakiyingi J, Quigley MA, et al. Inverse association between BCG immunisation and intestinal nematode infestation among HIV-1-positive indi-viduals in Uganda. *Lancet* 1999 Sep 18;354(9183):1000–1001.

12. Aaby P, Shaheen SO, Heyes CB, et al. Early BCG vaccination and reduction in atopy in Guinea-Bissau. *Clin Exp Allergy* 2000;30(5):644–650.

13. Cunha SS, Rodrigues LC, Pedrosa V, Dourado IM, Barreto ML, Pereira SM. Neonatal BCG protection against leprosy: a study in Manaus, Brazilian Ama-zon. *Lepr Rev* 2004;75:357–366.

14. Comstock GW, Edwards PQ. An American view of BCG vaccination, illus-trated by results of a controlled trial in Puerto Rico. *Dis Scand J Resp* 1972;53: 207–217.

15. Comstock GW, Woolpert SF, Livesay VT. Tuberculosis studies in Muscogee County, Georgia. *Public Health Rep* 1976;91(3):276–280.

16. Tuberculosis Prevention Trial. Trial of BCG vaccines in south India for tuber-culosis prevention. *Indian J Med Res* 1980;72(suppl):1–74.

17. Rosenthal SR, Loewinsohn E, Graham ML, Liveright D, Thorne MG, Johnson V. BCG vaccination against tuberculosis in Chicago. A twenty-year study sta-tistically analyzed. *Pedriatics* 1961;6:622–641.

18. Aronson JD. Protective vaccination against tuberculosis with special reference to BCG vaccination. *Am Rev Tuberc* 1948;58:255–281.

19. Hart PDA, Sutherland I. BCG and vole bacillus vaccines in the prevention of tuberculosis in adolescence and early adult life. Final report to the Medical Re-search Council. *Br Med J* 1977;2:293–295.

20. ten Dam HG, Hitze KL. Determining the prevalence of tuberculosis infection in populations with non-specific tuberculin sensitivity. *Bull World Health Organ* 1980;58(3):475–483.

21. Springett VH, Sutherland I. A re-examination of the variations in the efficacy of BCG vaccination against tuberculosis in clinical trials. *Tuber Lung Dis* 1994; 75(3):227–233.

22. Blin P, Delolme HG, Heyraud JD, Charpak Y, Sentilhes L. Evaluation of the protective effect of BCG vaccination by a case-control study in Yayounde, Cameroon. *Tubercle* 1986;67:283–288.

23. Costa MCN, Mota ELA, Pinto LLS. Efeito protetor do BCG intradérmico na meningite tuberculosa. *Bol Sanit Panam* 1991;110(1):26–32.

24. Camargos PAM, Guimarães MDC, Antunes CMF. Risk assessment for acquiring meningitis tuberculosis among children not vaccinated with BCG: a case-control study. *Int J Epidemiol* 1988;17(1):193–197.
25. Miceli I, Kantor IN, Colaiacovo D, et al. Evaluation of the effectiveness of BCG vaccination using the case-control method in Buenos Aires, Argentina. *Int J Epidemiol* 1988;17(3):629–634.
26. Mynt TT, Wint H, Aye H, Kyaw TO. Case-control study on evaluation of BCG vaccination of newborns in Rangoon, Burma. *Ann Trop Paed* 1987;7:159–166.
27. Packe GE, Innes JA. Protective effect of BCG vaccination in infant Asians: a case-control study. *Arch Dis Child* 1988;63:277–281.
28. Sirinavin S, Chotpitayasunondh T, Suwanjutha S, Sunakorn P, Chantarojanasiriet T. Protective efficacy of neonatal Bacillus Calmette-Guerin vaccination against tuberculosis. *Pediatr Infect Dis* 1991;10:359–365.
29. Patel A, Schofield F, Siskind V, Abrahams E, Parkeret J. Case-control evaluation of a school-age BCG vaccination programme in subtropical Australia. *Bull World Health Org* 1991;69(4):425–433.
30. Rodrigues L, Gill ON, Smith PG. BCG vaccination in the first year of life protects children of Indian subcontinent ethnic origin against tuberculosis in England. *J Epidemiol Community Health* 1991;45:78–80.
31. Orege PA, Fine PEM, Lucas SB, Obura M, Okelo C, Okuku P. Case-control study of BCG vaccination as a risk factor for leprosy and tuberculosis in Western Kenya. *Int J Lepr* 1992;61(4):542–549.
32. Shapiro C, Cook N, Evans D, et al. A case-control study of BCG and chilhood tuberculosis in Cali, Colombia. *Int J Epidemiol* 1985;14(3):441–446.
33. Young TK, Hershfield ES. A case-control study to evaluate the effectiveness of mass neonatal BCG vaccination among Canadian Indians. *Am J Public Health* 1986;76(7):783–786.
34. Zodpey SP, Maldhure BR, Shrikhande SN, Tiwari RR. Effectiveness of bacillus of Calmette-Guerin (BCG) vaccination against tuberculous meningitis: a case-control study. *J Indian Med Assoc* 1996;94(9):338–340.
35. Zodpey SP, Shrikhande SN, Maldhure BR, Vasudeo ND, Kulkarni SW. Effectiveness of bacillus Calmette Guerin (BCG) vaccination in the prevention of childhood pulmonary tuberculosis: a case-control study in Nagpur, India. *Southeast Asian J Trop Med Public Health* 1998;29(2):285–288.
36. Wunsch Filho V, de Castilho EA, Rodrigues LC, Huttly SR. Effectiveness of BCG vaccination against tuberculous meningitis: a case-control study in Sao Paulo, Brazil. *Bull World Health Organ* 1990;68(1):69–74.
37. Thilothammal N, Krishnamurthy PV, Runyan DK, Banu K. Does BCG vaccine prevent tuberculous meningitis? *Arch Dis Child* 1996;74:144–147.
38. Bhat GJ, Diwan VK, Chintu C, Kabika M, Masona J. HIV, BCG and TB in children: a case study in Lusaka, Zambia. *J Trop Pediatr* 1993;39(4):219–223.
39. Arbeláez MP, Kenrad NE, Muñoz A. BCG vaccine effectiveness in preventing tuberculosis and its interaction with human immunodeficiency virus infection. *Int J of Epidemiol* 2000;29:1085–1091.
40. Colditz GA, Berkey CS, Mosteller F, et al. The efficacy of bacillus Calmette-Guerin vaccination of newborns and infants in the prevention of tuberculosis: meta-analyses of the published literature. *Pediatrics* 1995;96(1 Pt 1):29–35.
41. Colditz GA, Brewer TF, Berkey CS, et al. Efficacy of BCG vaccine in the prevention of tuberculosis. Meta-analysis of the published literature. *JAMA* 1994;271(9):698–702.

42. Rodrigues LC, Diwan VK, Wheeler JG. Protective effect of BCG against tuber-culous meningitis and miliary tuberculosis: a meta-analysis. *Int J Epidemiol* 1993;22(6):1154–1158.
43. Smith KC, Starke JR. Bacille Calmette-Guerin vaccine. In: Plotkin SA, Orenstein WA eds. *Vaccines*. 4th ed. Philadelphia: WB Saunders Company, 2004:179–209.
44. Fine PE. Vaccines and vaccination. In: Reichman LB, Hershfield ES, eds. *Tuberculosis: A Comprehensive and International Approach*. New York: Marcel Dekker 2000.
45. Fine PE, Vynnycky E. The effect of heterologous immunity upon the apparent efficacy of (e.g. BCG) vaccines. *Vaccine* 1998;16(20):1923–1928.
46. Luelmo F. BCG vaccination. *Am Rev Respir Dis* 1982;125:70–72.
47. Wilson ME, Fineberg HV, Colditz G. Geographic latitude and the efficacy of bacillus Calmette-Guerin vaccine. *Clin Infect Dis* 1995;20:982–991.
48. Sterne JA, Rodrigues LC, Guedes IN. Does the efficacy of BCG decline with time since vaccination? *Int J Tuber Lung Dis* 1998;2(3):200–207.
49. Aronson NE, Santosham M, Comstock GW. Long-term efficacy of BCG vac-cine in American Indians and Alaska Natives: a 60 year follow up study. *JAMA* 2004;291:2086–2091.
50. Barreto M, Cunha SS, Pereira SM, Genser B, Hijjar MA, Ichihara MY, Brito SC, Dourado I, Cruz A, Sant'Ana C, Rodrigues LC. Neonatal BCG protects chil-dren and young adults against all forms of tuberculosis in Brazil. *Int J Tuber Lung Dis* 2005;9:1171–1173.
51. WHO. Global tuberculosis programme and global programme on vaccines—statement on BCG revaccination for the prevention of tuberculosis. *Wkly Epidemiol Rec* 1995;70:229–231.
52. Lugosi L. Results of the BCG vaccination in Hungary since 1929: evaluation of preventive and immunotherapeutic effectiveness. *Orv Hetil.* 1998;139(26): 1563–1570.
53. Sepulveda RL, Parcha C, Sorensen RU. Case-control study of the efficacy of BCG immunization against pulmonary tuberculosis in young adults in Santi-ago, Chile. *Tuber Lung Dis* 1993;73(6):372–377.
54. Tala-Heikkila MM, Tuominem JE, Tala EOJ. Bacillus Calmette-Guérin revacci-nation questionable with low tuberculosis incidence. *Am J Respir Care Med* 1998;157:1324–1327.
55. Karonga Prevention Trial Group. Randomised controlled trial of single BCG, repeated BCG, or combined BCG and killed *Mycobacterium leprae* vaccine for prevention of leprosy and tuberculosis in Malawi [see comments]. *Lancet* 1996; 348(9019):17–24.
56. Rodrigues LC, Pereira SM, Cunha SS, Genser B, Ichihara MY, de Brito SC, Hijjar MA, Dourado I, Cruz AA, Sant'Ana C, Bierrenbach AL, Barreto ML. Effect of BCG revaccination on incidence of tuberculosis in school-aged chil-dren in Brazil: the BCG-REVAC cluster-randomised trial. *Lancet.* 2005;366 (9493):1290–1295.
57. Cunha SS. BCG effectiveness against leprosy among school children in Ama-zon Region, Northern Brazil [PhD thesis]. London School of Hygiene and Tropical Medicine. University of London, UK, 2004.
58. Karalliedde S, Katugaha LP, Uragoda CG. Tuberculin response of Sri Lankan children after BCG vaccination at birth. *Tubercle* 1987;68(1):33–38.
59. Pereira SM, Dourado MI, Barreto ML, et al. Sensitivity and specificity of BCG scar reading in Brazil. *Int J Tuber and Lung Dis* 2001;5(11):1067–1070.

60. Pereira SM, Bierrenbach AL, Dourado I, et al. Sensibility and speficity of the BCG scar reading. *Rev Saude Publica* 2003;37(2):254–259.
61. Grindulis H, Baynham MI, Scott PH, Thompson RA, Wharton BA. Tuberculin response two years after BCG vaccination at birth. *Arch Dis Child* 1984;59(7): 614–619.
62. Young TK, Mirdad S. Determinants of tuberculin sensitivity in a child population covered by mass BCG vaccination. *Tuber Lung Dis* 1992;73(2):94–100.
63. Sterne JA, Fine PE, Ponnighaus JM, Sibanda F, Munthali M, Glynn JR. Does bacille Calmette-Guerin scar size have implications for protection against tuberculosis or leprosy? *Tuber Lung Dis* 1996;77(2):117–123.
64. Aggarwal A, Dutta AK. Timing and dose of BCG vaccination in infants as assessed by postvaccination tuberculin sensitivity. *Indian Pediatr* 1995;32(6): 635–639.
65. Bierrenbach AL, Cunha SS, Barreto ML, et al. Tuberculin reactivity in a population of schoolchildren with high BCG coverage. *Rev Panam Salud Publica* 2003;13(5):285–292.
66. Brewer TF, Colditz GA. Relationship between bacille Calmette-Guerin (BCG) strains and the efficacy of BCG vaccine in the prevention of tuberculosis. *Clin Infect Dis* 1995;20(1):126–135.
67. Wang L, Turner MO, Elwood RK, Schulzer M, Fitzgerald JM. A meta-analysis of the effect of bacille Calmette Guerin vaccination on tuberculin skin test measurements. *Thorax* 2002;57:804–809.
68. Cunha SS, Dourado I, Barreto ML, et al. Design of the leprosy component of the Brazilian BCG revaccination trial for assessing BCG effectiveness against leprosy in schoolchildren. *Int J Lepr Other Mycobact Dis* 2004;72:8–15.
69. Cunha SS. *A trial of BCG vaccine effectiveness against leprosy among school children in Manaus, Northern Brazil.* London: London School of Hygiene and Tropical Medicine, 2003.
70. Abel L, Cua VV, Oberti J, et al. Leprosy and BCG in southern Vietnam [letter; comment] [see comments]. *Lancet* 1990;335(8704):1536.
71. Lombardi C, Pedrazzani ES, Pedrazzani JC, Filho PF, Zicker F. Protective efficacy of BCG against leprosy in Sao Paulo. *Bull Pan Am Health Organ* 1996;30(1): 24–30.
72. Zodpey SP, Bansod BS, Shrikhande SN, Maldhure BR, Kulkarni SW. Protective effect of bacillus Calmette Guerin (BCG) against leprosy: a population-based case-control study in Nagpur, India. *Lepr Rev* 1999;70(3):287–294.
73. Zodpey SP, Ambadekar NN, Thakur A. Effectiveness of bacillus Calmette Guerin (BCG) vaccination in the prevention of leprosy: a population-based case-control study in Yavatmal District, India. *Public Health* 2005;119:209–216.
74. Convit J, Smith PG, Zuniga M, et al. BCG vaccination protects against leprosy in Venezuela: a case-control study. *Int J Lepr Other Mycobact Dis* 1993;61(2): 185–191.
75. Fine P, Ponnighaus JM, Maine N, Clarkson JA. Protective efficacy of BCG against leprosy in northern Malawi. *Lancet* 1986;30:499–504.
76. Muliyil J, Nelson KE, Diamond EL. Effect of BCG on the risk of leprosy in an endemic area: a case control study [see comments]. *Int J Lepr Other Mycobact Dis* 1991;59(2):229–236.

77. Thuc NV, Abel L, Lap VD, Oberti J, Lagrange PH. Protective effect of BCG against leprosy and its subtypes: a case-control study in southern Vietnam. *Int J Lepr Other Mycobact Dis* 1994;62(4):532–538.
78. Bertolli J, Pangi C, Frerichs R, Halloran ME. A case-control study of the effectiveness of BCG vaccine for preventing leprosy in Yangon, Myanmar. *Int J Epidemiol* 1997;26(4):888–896.
79. Smith WC. What is the best way to use BCG to protect against leprosy: when, for whom, and how often? *Int J Lepr Other Mycobact Dis* 2004;72:48–49.
80. Cunha SS, Rodrigues LC, Duppre NC. Current strategy for leprosy control in Brazil: time to pursue alternative preventive strategies? *Rev Panam Salud Publica* 2004;16:362–365.
81. Lotte A, Wasz-Hockert O, Poisson N, Dumitrescu N, Verron M, Couvet E. BCG complications. *Adv Tuber Res* 1984;21:107–193.
82. Moss WJ, Clements J, Halsey N. Immunization of children at risk of infection with human immunodeficiency virus. *Bull WHO* 2003;81:61–70.
83. Dourado I, Rios MH, Pereira SM, et al. Rates of adverse reactions to first and second doses of BCG vaccination: results of a large community trial in Brazil schoolchildren. *Int J Tuber Lung Dis* 2003;7(4): 399–402.
84. Joint Tuberculosis Committee. Control and prevention of tuberculosis in the United Kingdom: code of practice 2000. *Thorax* 2000;55:887–901.
85. World Health Organization. BCG vaccine. WHO position paper. *Wkly Epidemiol Rec* 2004;79(4):27–38.
86. Diel R, Seidler A, Nienhaus A, Rush-Gerdes S, Niemann S. Ocupational risk of tuberculosis transmission. *Respir Res* 2005;6:1–35.
87. Ginsberg AM. What's new in tuberculosis vaccines? *Bull World Health Organ* 2002;80(6):483–488.
88. von Reyn CF, Vuola JM. New vaccines for the prevention of tuberculosis. *Clin Infect Dis* 2002;35(4):465–474.
89. Brennan M. The tuberculosis vaccine challenge. *Tuberculosis* 2005;85(1–2):7–12.
90. Snider DEJ. Ethical issues in tuberculosis vaccine trials. *Clin Infect Dis* 2000; 30(3:S):271–275.

VACCINATION SAFETY

Lucia Helena de Oliveira, MSc,[1] *Carlos Castillo-Solórzano,*
MD, MPH,[2] *M. Carolina Danovaro-Holliday, MD, MSc,*[3]
José Peña-Ruz, Pharm Chem PhD,[4] *and Jon Kim Andrus, MD*[5]

INTRODUCTION

The prevention of infectious diseases through immunization ranks as one of the finest achievements in public health. As vaccine-preventable diseases become less visible through effective vaccination programs, more attention is paid to clinical symptoms that appear following the administration of a vaccine, a phenomenon that is referred to as "events supposedly attributable to vaccination or immunization" (ESAVI) *(1)*.

For the most part, vaccines are administered to large groups of infants who are more vulnerable to diseases and developmental problems, such as hearing loss. Moreover, the majority of vaccines are administered during the initial years of life. The temporal relationship between the onset of developmental problems and the administration of vaccines increases the likelihood that developmental problems may be viewed as being caused by the vaccine. Therefore, vaccine safety is of critical importance. Most childhood vaccinations may result in mild adverse events, including local reactions such as redness and swelling at the injection site. Rare and more serious reactions, such as allergic reactions, also can occur. There may be allergic reactions to the biological components, to chemical products used

[1] Regional Advisor on New Vaccines, Immunization Unit, Pan American Health Organization.

[2] Regional Advisor on Vaccines and Immunization, Pan American Health Organization.

[3] Technical Officer, Immunization Unit, Pan American Health Organization.

[4] Technical Officer, Technology and Health Services Delivery, Essential Medicines, Vaccines and Health Technologies Unit, Pan American Health Organization.

[5] Lead Technical Advisor, Immunization Unit, Pan American Health Organization.

in the vaccine manufacturing process, or, in the case of live vaccines, to the virulent organisms. Any serious event should be thoroughly investigated to rule out or confirm the vaccine as the cause *(1–6)*.

Every effort should be made to guarantee the use of high-quality vaccines and safe injection practices by strengthening ESAVI monitoring *(7)*. Beneficiaries need to believe that the services being provided to them are justified and delivered with the highest possible standards. Communication should also be an essential priority of national immunization programs. Effective messages should be delivered to families at the same time that the services are provided *(1, 8)*.

EVENTS SUPPOSEDLY ATTRIBUTABLE TO VACCINATION OR IMMUNIZATION

An adverse event to a biological product may be simply defined as an event associated with the use of the biological product. Adverse events include any side effect, injury, toxicity, sensitivity reaction, or significant failure to generate immune response *(9)*. In the Region of the Americas, the term ESAVIs refers to all adverse events following immunization *(1)*.

Most events associated with vaccination are local reactions, fever, and generalized malaise and may be categorized as mild (Table 1) *(10–12)*. A vaccine is designed to provide protection against infection by inducing cellular and humoral immunity in the person vaccinated. A mild reaction such as redness and swelling, and low-grade fever, can all be part of the normal immune response. Certain components of the vaccine (for example, aluminum adjuvant, antibiotics, or preservatives) can also contribute to these events *(2, 4)*.

In contrast to mild events, severe events are very rare (Table 2). Almost all serious events (for example, seizures, thrombocytopenia, episodes of hypotonia and hyporesponsiveness, and persistent, inconsolable crying) are characterized by spontaneous remission and do not lead to sequelae. Although anaphylaxis, defined as hypersensitivity to any component of the vaccine resulting from sensitization following prior contact with the causative agent, can be fatal, it does not leave sequelae if treated in a timely manner. Encephalopathy is cited as a rare event associated with measles and DTP vaccines *(2, 4)*.

INVESTIGATION OF ESAVIs

Because public confidence is at stake, proper monitoring of ESAVIs requires rapid and accurate detection, investigation, assessment, management, and

TABLE 1. Rates of mild events attributable to vaccination.

Vaccine	Clinical signs		
	Local reaction (pain, swelling, redness)	Fever	Irritability, malaise, and nonspecific symptoms
Bacille Calmette-Guérin (BCG)[a]	Common[b]	—	—
Diphtheria, pertussis, tetanus (DPT)[c]	Up to 50%	Up to 50%	Up to 60%
Hepatitis B	Up to 30% in adults Up to 5% in children	1%–6%	Infrequent[d]
Haemophilus influenzae type b (Hib)	5–15%	2%–10%	Rare
Measles, mumps, rubella (MMR)	Up to 10%	Up to 5%	Up to 5%
Oral polio vaccine (OPV)	None	Less than 1%	Less than 1%[e]
Tetanus (TT), tetanus, diphtheria (Td)	Up to 10%[f]	Up to 10%	Up to 25%

[a] Local reactogenicity varies from vaccine to vaccine, depending on the strain and number of viable bacilli.
[b] Local lymphadenopathy is associated.
[c] For the whole-cell pertussis vaccine. The rates of local reaction for acellular pertussis vaccine are lower.
[d] Children vaccinated against DPT and hepatitis B generally do not have more reactions than children who only receive DPT.
[e] Diarrhea, headache, and muscle pain are the usual complaints.
[f] The rate of local events is likely to increase from 50% to 85% with subsequent booster doses.

Sources: World Health Organization, Department of Vaccines and Biologicals; *Supplementary information on vaccine safety.* Part 2: *Background rates of adverse events following immunization.* Geneva: WHO; 2000 (WHO/V&B/00.36); Greenberg DP. *Pediatric experience with recombinant hepatitis B vaccines and relevant safety and immunogenicity studies.* Pediatr Infect Dis J. 1993 May;12(5):438–45. Review; and Pan American Health Organization. Control of Diphtheria, Pertussis, Tetanus, *Haemophilus influenzae* type b and Hepatitis B Field Guide. Scientific and Technical Publication No. 604. Washington, DC: PAHO, 2005.

prevention *(17)*. It is essential to develop a communication plan to inform the public about any incidents that might occur *(1, 8, 18)*.

Adverse events that particularly merit investigation are:

• Severe events—those that require hospitalization, are potentially life-threatening, cause disability, or have fatal outcomes.
• Events that occur in clusters.
• Events related to the program (programmatic errors).
• Rumors that may seriously undermine confidence of the public served.

CAUSALITY

As mentioned earlier, events that are only temporally related may often occur following vaccination. Thus, before declaring a causal relationship

TABLE 2. Time between vaccination and event onset, and rates of severe events attributable to vaccination.

Vaccine	Event	Time between vaccination and event onset	Rates per 1,000,000 doses
BCG	Suppurative lymphadenitis	2–6 months	100–1,000
	BCG osteitis	1–12 months	1–700
DPT	Persistent, inconsolable crying for more than 3 hours	0–24 hours	1,000–60,000
	Seizures	0–2 days	570[a]
	Hypotonic-hyporesponsive episode (HHE)	0–24 hours	570
	Anaphylaxis	0–1 hour	20
	Encephalopathy	0–3 days	0–1
Hepatitis B	Anaphylaxis	0–1 hour	1–2
	Guillain-Barré syndrome (plasma-derived vaccine)	0–6 weeks	5
Hib	No known severe event	—	—
Measles/MMR[b]	Febrile seizures	5–12 days	333
	Thrombocytopenia	15–35 days	33
	Anaphylaxis	0–1 hour	1–50
	Aseptic meningitis	18–34 days	0.002–1,160 depending on the strain
Oral polio vaccine(OPV)	Vaccine-associated paralytic polio (VAPP)	4–40 days	Less than 1[c]
TT/Td	Neuritis of the brachial plexus	2–28 days	5–10
	Anaphylaxis	0–1 hour	1–6
	Sterile abscess	1–6 weeks	6–10
Yellow fever	Post-vaccination encephalitis	7–21 days	500–4,000 in infants under 6 months of age 5–20[d]
	Allergic/anaphylactic reaction	0–1 hour	

[a] The seizures are mainly of febrile origin, and the rate depends on individual and family history and age, with a lower risk in infants under 4 months of age.

[b] There are no reactions (except for anaphylaxis) when immunity is present (~90% of those who receive a second dose). Febrile seizures are unlikely in children over 6 years of age.

[c] The risk of VAPP is higher with the first OPV dose (1 per 1,400,000–3,400,000 doses) than with subsequent doses and contacts, 1 per 5,900,000–13,030,000 and 1 per 6,700,000 doses, respectively.

[d] Isolated cases, without a denominator, hinder evaluation of the rate in older children and adults, but are very rare (less than 1 case per 8,000,000 doses).

Sources: World Health Organization, Department of Vaccines and Biologicals; *Supplementary information on vaccine safety. Part 2: Background rates of adverse events following immunization.* Geneva: WHO; 2000 (WHO/V&B/00.36); de Oliveira LH, Struchiner CJ. Vaccine-associated paralytic poliomyelitis in Brazil, 1989–1995. *Rev Panam Salud Publica.* 2000;7(4):219–24; de Oliveira LH, Struchiner CJ. Vaccine-associated paralytic poliomyelitis: a retrospective cohort study of acute flaccid paralyses in Brazil. *Int J Epidemiol.* 2000; 29(4):757–763; Centers for Disease Control and Prevention. Poliomyelitis Prevention in the United States: Introduction of a Sequential Vaccination Schedule of Inactivated Poliovirus Vaccine Followed by Oral Poliovirus Vaccine; Recommendations of the Advisory Committee on Immunization Practices (ACIP). *MMWR.* 1997; 46(RR-3); and Centers for Disease Control and Prevention. NIP answers your questions: Polio. *What is the incidence of vaccine associated paralytic polio (VAPP) in the developing world?* http://www.cdc.gov/nip/faqs/polio-faqs.htm#OPV; World Health Organization. *Wkly Epidemiol Rec.* 2001;76(45):345–356.

between an adverse event and a vaccine, well-designed studies should be conducted to test causality. In some situations the investigation may prove to be inconclusive, usually because the number of cases is small or other data are insufficient *(2, 19–21)*.

Several questions should be asked when evaluating an adverse event *(20)*:

- What has been the previous experience with the vaccine? How many people have been vaccinated with the vaccine in question? How many people have experienced similar events?
- Is there an alternative etiological candidate that causes the same type of event?
- Have these individuals received the vaccine before and, if so, did they experience an adverse event?
- Do persons with adverse events have a medical history or genetic susceptibility that would affect the risk of an adverse event occurring as a result of vaccination?
- Did the adverse event occur within the time frame in which causality is scientifically plausible?
- Is this adverse event part of a cluster of events that are associated with defined vaccine lots?
- Do the characteristics of this adverse event permit laboratory testing to support the hypothesis?
- Did the event resolve rapidly? Was it irreversible? Was treatment required?

In the case of ESAVI clusters, constructing an algorithm may facilitate evaluating and explaining the cluster *(1)* (Figure 1).

FINAL CLASSIFICATION FOLLOWING AN ESAVI INVESTIGATION

Data from the investigation should be analyzed to classify the event in one of three categories *(1)*:

1. Not related to vaccination,
2. Related to the vaccination, or
3. Inconclusive.

When the Event Is Not Related to Vaccination

These are events that occur following vaccination, but are not caused by it. The relation between the occurrence of the event and the vaccination is totally random and is simply *coincidental* with the vaccination. The event

FIGURE 1. Algorithm for evaluating causality in an event supposedly attributable to vaccination or immunization cluster.

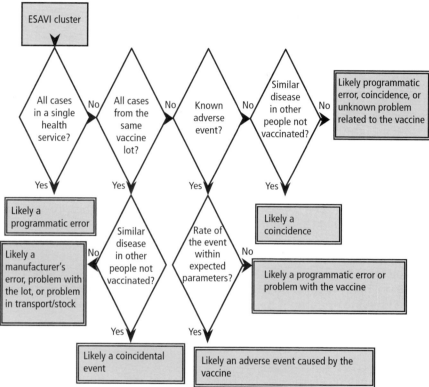

Source: Pan American Health Organization. Vaccine Safety Modules. Washington, D.C.: PAHO, 2006 (in process of publication).

could have occurred even if the individual had not received the vaccine. A useful approach to justify the conclusion that the event is coincidental is to show that similar events occur in persons who have not been immunized. It is important to use sound methodologies. Studies should be designed to determine if the frequency of the event in question is statistically different in the vaccinated group versus the unvaccinated one. Such studies should be designed to minimize all biases, especially selection bias between comparison groups (1, 20).

Although the ESAVI may have been unrelated to the vaccination, adequate monitoring by a physician may be indicated to provide the necessary care regardless of the etiology (1).

When the Event Is Related to the Vaccination

The Event Is Related to Operational Aspects of the Program (Programmatic Error)

Programmatic errors in the management of the storage, reconstitution, handling, or administration of the vaccine may contribute to the occurrence of adverse events. The vaccinator must take all precautions to prevent events caused by "programmatic errors." In these cases, the event is associated with human error, rather than errors inherent in the vaccine or technology. They can usually be prevented by training personnel, supervising the administration of vaccines, and ensuring an adequate supply of equipment for administering safe injections (1, 22–27).

A programmatic error can lead to a cluster of events. Improperly administered vaccinations can result in abscesses or other blood-borne infections. Toxic shock syndrome is a serious, life-threatening adverse event caused by improper handling of the vaccine vial once the product has been reconstituted. The vial becomes contaminated with bacterial overgrowth. Staphylococcal overgrowth is one of the most common causes of toxic shock syndrome, as the bacteria produce a toxin that causes vascular collapse (28). Vaccinating infants from such a contaminated vial could result in many deaths shortly after injection. Programmatic errors are caused by one or more of the following situations (1, 4, 29–32):

- Improper dosage.
- Improper method of administration.
- Reuse of disposable syringes.
- Unsafe use of needles and syringes, such as not adhering to a sterile technique, resulting in contamination of the vaccine or diluent.
- Failure to check the packaging to guarantee the sterility of needles and syringes.
- Reconstitution of the vaccines with the wrong diluent or diluent amount.
- Substitution of vaccines or diluents with drugs or other substances.
- Improper storage of vaccines and syringes.
- Use of vaccines and syringes after the expiration date.

The Event Is Related to the Vaccination Itself

This type of event implies a causal relation between the event and the vaccination. As previously mentioned, the most common reactions are usually mild and expected, while serious reactions are extremely rare. A vaccination-related event is an event caused or precipitated by the inherent properties of the vaccine or its components (1, 2, 4, 20, 32).

- Intrinsic reactions—reactions caused by the patient's immune response to the biological antigen used in the vaccine.

- Extrinsic reactions—reactions caused by the patient's response to other components in the formulation. These are reactions of the patient's immune system to any of the other components used in the vaccine formulation, such as:
  1. Resuspension agents, such as water or saline solution.
  2. Preservatives, such as thimerosal.
  3. Stabilizers, such as sorbitol and hydrolyzed gelatin (in the MMR vaccine).
  4. Adjuvants, such as aluminum salts.
  5. Residue from culture media.
  6. Antibiotics, such as Neomycin and Streptomycin (inactivated polio vaccine, varicella vaccine).
- Factors related to the host—event caused by genetic susceptibility, anxiety, or pain from the injection, not the vaccine.
- Unacceptable vaccine quality—divergence from vaccine-licensing parameters, such as an increase in the concentration of the virus.

When the Investigation Is Inconclusive

In some situations, even after an exhaustive investigation (epidemiological, clinical, and laboratory) it is not possible to determine causality. In that case, the interested parties should be notified of the findings and explained why a conclusion could not be reached (1, 2, 32).

A similar classification and assessment of causality is used in the United States (3). An ESAVI is classified by frequency (common or rare), extent (local or systemic), severity (hospitalization, disability, death), causality, and preventability (intrinsic to vaccine, faulty production, faulty administration). Following that classification, ESAVIs can be divided as:

- Vaccine-induced—due to the intrinsic characteristics of the vaccine preparation and the individual's response to the vaccine.
- Vaccine-potentiated—the event would have occurred anyway, but was precipitated by the vaccination.
- Programmatic error—event due to technical errors in vaccine storage, preparation, handling, or administration.
- Coincidental—the reported event was not caused by vaccination, but happened by chance occurrence, or due to underlying illness.

SPECIAL CONDITIONS FOR VACCINATION

Pregnancy

The antigens in inactivated vaccines are, by definition, not live. They do not replicate. Therefore, inactivated antigens cannot infect the fetus during pregnancy. Inactivated vaccines are indicated for pregnant women and vaccination should follow existing guidelines *(33)*.

In general, antigens in live vaccines must replicate in order to confer enhanced immunity. Even though in most cases no fetal adverse events have been observed, live vaccines should be generally avoided during pregnancy to prevent the vaccine from being temporally associated with some event in the newborn. Causality in such events is extremely difficult to prove. In special situations where the risk of contracting vaccine-preventable diseases is high, the possibility of vaccination of pregnant women should be considered, for example in yellow fever endemic areas *(6, 33)*.

Vaccines in pregnancy can be categorized as vaccines with no contraindications, vaccines recommended in special circumstances, and vaccines that are contraindicated (Table 3).

Immunosuppression

Live vaccines can cause severe reactions in immunocompromised patients. Replication of the vaccine virus has the potential of going unchecked in an immunocompromised vaccine recipient, potentially causing disease. Hence, immunocompromised patients such as those with leukemia or lymphoma should not receive live vaccines *(37, 38)*.

Inactivated vaccines are generally safe for use in immunocompromised patients because the antigen cannot replicate. However, the immunogenicity of inactivated vaccines may be decreased in these patients.

Some drugs, such as those used in chemotherapy, or prolonged treatment with corticoids, can produce immunosuppression. Patients receiving these drugs should not receive live vaccines (for example the OPV vaccine). In general, if chemotherapy is suspended for at least three months, patients can again receive live vaccines *(37, 39, 40)*. With corticosteroid therapy, the dose and duration of the therapy should be considered. If patients receive corticoids at the dose of 2 mg/kg/day, or 20 mg/day, for more than 14 days, the contraindication should be maintained.

HIV Infection

With some notable exceptions, immunization is generally safe and beneficial for HIV-infected persons. Routine screening for HIV status before vaccination is not recommended. Patients with HIV may be asymptomatic or exhibit symptoms ranging from mildly to severely immunocompromised. In general, the rules for these patients are the same as those in the paragraph above—live vaccines should generally be avoided (Table 4). Most HIV-infected children have the capacity to mount both cellular and

TABLE 3. Vaccinating pregnant women.

Vaccine	Recommendation
No contraindications	
Influenza	Pregnant women, after their first trimester of pregnancy, should receive inactivated influenza vaccine during the flu season. If a pregnant woman has a medical condition that would imply a greater risk of complications from influenza, she should be vaccinated at any stage of gestation.
Tetanus/Diphtheria	All women with an incomplete tetanus/diphtheria series should be vaccinated with Td at their first contact with prenatal services.
Indicated in special circumstances	
Anthrax	Vaccination is recommended if there is exposure occupationally or exposure through bioterrorism. Contact with human cases does not require immunization.
Cholera	There is no specific information on the safety of cholera vaccine during pregnancy. The decision to use this vaccine should be made on a case-by-case basis.
Hepatitis A	If a pregnant woman is at high risk for contracting hepatitis A, vaccination could be considered.
Hepatitis B	Hepatitis B virus infection in pregnancy can cause serious disease in the mother and chronic infection in the fetus. Hepatitis B vaccination is recommended in pregnant women at risk of hepatitis B virus infection.
Japanese encephalitis (JE)	There is no specific information on the safety of JE vaccine during pregnancy and the theoretical risk that JE vaccine poses to the fetus is unknown. JE vaccine is not routinely administered to pregnant women. If a pregnant woman must travel to an endemic area, the vaccine should be administered only if the perceived benefit outweighs the risk.
Meningococcus	Studies have shown meningococcus vaccine to be safe and effective in pregnancy. High levels of antibodies have been found in the umbilical cord. The antibody titles decline in the first months of life without affecting the response to subsequent vaccination.
Plague	The effect of this vaccine on the developing fetus is unknown. The mother should be instructed in practices that reduce the risk of exposure. Only if the potential benefit outweighs the risk to the fetus should this vaccine be administered.
Pneumococcus	The safety of this vaccine during the first trimester of pregnancy has not been evaluated. However, adverse events have not been reported in newborns born to mothers who were inadvertently vaccinated.

(Table continues on next page)

TABLE 3. (Continued).

Vaccine	Recommendation
Oral polio vaccine	Although adverse events have not been documented in pregnant women or their infants, polio vaccination should be avoided during pregnancy. If a pregnant woman requires immediate immunization, the general recommendations for adults should be followed.
Poliovirus vaccine inactivated	There are no contraindications for pregnancy or breast-feeding.
Rabies	There is no evidence of fetal anomalies associated with rabies vaccine. If there is a high risk of rabies exposure, vaccination during pregnancy should be considered.
Yellow fever	Pregnant women should not be vaccinated against yellow fever or travel to yellow fever endemic areas. If a pregnant woman must travel to an endemic area, vaccination should be considered only if the risk of yellow fever in that area is very high.
Contraindicated	
BCG	Although no association between the vaccine and adverse events in the fetus or newborn has been reported, this vaccine should not be administered during pregnancy.
Rubella[a]	Avoiding rubella vaccination during pregnancy is recommended to prevent implicating the vaccine in any event that might occur. However, there is no need to advise women on avoiding pregnancy after receiving the rubella vaccine. Also, if a pregnant woman is inadvertently vaccinated, interrupting pregnancy should not be recommended.
Measles	The virus in the measles vaccine does not cross the placenta and, thus, cannot infect the fetus. However, as with rubella vaccine, measles vaccine should not be administered to pregnant women to prevent implicating the vaccine in potential complications of pregnancy.
Mumps	If administered in conjunction with the vaccines for measles and rubella (MMR vaccine), the recommendations for the other two vaccines should be followed.
Smallpox	This vaccine should not be administered to pregnant women. Fetal infection has been reported following primary immunization, although there is no evidence of congenital malformations. The use of specific gamma-globulin (0.3 ml/kg) is indicated before exposure to the virus or if the vaccine has been inadvertently administered to a pregnant woman.
Varicella	Varicella (chickenpox) vaccine should not be administered to pregnant women. Also, avoiding conception for four weeks after vaccination is advisable.

[a] No cases of congenital rubella syndrome have been detected in newborns from women vaccinated inadvertently with rubella vaccine during pregnancy (*34–36*).

Source: Ávila ML, Castillo-Solórzano C. Vacunación en la mujer embarazada. *Acta Pediátrica Costarricense* 2005;19(3).

TABLE 4. Guidelines for immunizing HIV-infected persons.

Vaccines that should continue to be offered routinely to all HIV-positive persons, both symptomatic and asymptomatic, according to the country's standard schedule:
- Diphtheria-pertussis-tetanus (DPT) vaccine.
- *Haemophilus influenzae* type b (Hib) vaccine.
- Tetanus toxoid and tetanus-diphtheria vaccines
  (including at childbearing age and pregnant women).

Vaccines that should continue to be offered routinely to HIV-positive children with some specific considerations:
- Measles-mumps-rubella (MMR) vaccine: MMR should be routinely administered to HIV-infected children unless they are severely immunosuppressed.[a] MMR should be administered as early in life as possible, according to the nationally recommended schedules. In an outbreak situation, HIV-infected (known or suspected) infants at increased risk of exposure to measles should receive a first dose at 6 months of age and a second at 9 months of age.
- Oral polio vaccine (OPV): OPV has not been found harmful when administered to asymptomatic HIV-positive children. However, if available, inactivated polio vaccine (IPV) is preferred, especially for symptomatic individuals. IPV is preferred for HIV-positive individuals and their household contacts due to the theoretical risk of OPV's neurovirulent effect on immunocompromised persons.
- Hepatitis B vaccine: Recombinant hepatitis B vaccines are safe to use and are recommended following the country schedule for non-HIV-infected individuals. Early immunization is especially important as the risk of becoming a chronic carrier is higher for HIV-infected persons than for uninfected ones. The immunological response may be poor among HIV-positive individuals but there is not enough information to provide firm recommendations on dosage at this time.

Vaccines that should NOT be given to symptomatic HIV-infected persons (i.e., AIDS patients):
- BCG: In persons known or suspected to be infected with HIV, BCG vaccine is contraindicated if the risk of tuberculosis is considered low. However, it can be recommended at birth or as soon as possible thereafter, following the country's schedule, if the risk of tuberculosis is high, since BCG will protect the infant against extrapulmonary forms of TB.
- Yellow fever vaccine: Where the risk of yellow fever is high, yellow fever vaccine may be considered for HIV-positive persons.
- Live attenuated typhoid vaccine.
- Varicella vaccine.

Vaccines to be considered for HIV-infected persons given their increased risk of disease:
- Pneumococcal.
- Influenza.

[a] Age-specific CD4 T-lymphocyte count indicating severe immunosuppression in HIV infection

Age	<12 months	1–5 years	≥6 years
CD4 count	<750† (0.75 × 10⁹/L)	<500† (0.50 × 10⁹/L)	<200† (0.20 × 10⁹/L)

† Or <15% of total lymphocytes.

Source: Pan American Health Organization. Guidelines for immunizing HIV infected persons. *EPI Newsletter* 2005;27(2): 6–7.

humoral immune responses during the first two years of life; decline in these two responses occurs during the next two years. However, severely ill HIV-infected persons should not be vaccinated with live vaccines. As with other causes of immunocompromise, the efficacy of immunization varies among HIV-infected individuals, and the proportion of responders declines with progression from HIV infection to AIDS. Nevertheless, HIV-infected individuals of any age who are well-controlled on combination anti-retroviral therapy (undetected or low viral load with good preservation of CD4 lymphocyte count) are likely to respond well to all vaccines *(41–46)*.

Issues related to thimerosal, a preservative used in some vaccines and other biologicals since the 1930s, are not addressed in this chapter. As explained in several publications, no association between thimerosal and autism or other neurodevelopmental disorders has been found. For further information on this topic, we refer the reader to reports from the Global Advisory Committee on Vaccine Safety *(47)*, United States Institute of Medicine *(48)*, and PAHO's update on thimerosal and autism *(49)*.

CONCLUSIONS AND RECOMMENDATIONS

New vaccines are continually being added to the immunization schedules for children and adults, increasing the probability that adverse events may coincide with vaccination. Adequate conditions for vaccination, from the quality of vaccine production to vaccine administration, must be maintained and continually monitored through an ESAVI monitoring system. It is of critical importance for the immunization program to ensure that vaccines will not pose additional risks due to programmatic errors in which one or more vaccination standards have not been met. Adverse events must be monitored and aggressively evaluated as they occur. Systems should be strengthened to allow for accurate assessment of causality. Health workers in immunization programs should be very well trained in all aspects of safe vaccination and, above all, in methodologies to thoroughly investigate adverse events and to communicate their findings to the public. "It is much easier to create doubt and damage a vaccine's reputation than it is to restore it" *(50)*.

References

1. Pan American Health Organization. Vaccine Safety Modules. Washington, DC: PAHO, 2006 (in press).
2. World Health Organization. Surveillance of adverse events following immunization: field guide for managers of immunization programmes. Geneva: WHO, 1993. (WHO/EPI/TRAM/93.2).

3. Centers for Disease Control and Prevention. Update: Vaccine Side Effects, Adverse Reactions, Contraindications, and Precautions; Recommendations of the Advisory Committee on Immunization Practices (ACIP). *MMWR* 1996; 45(RR-12).

4. World Health Organization, Department of Vaccines and Biologicals; Supplementary information on vaccine safety. Part 2: Background rates of adverse events following immunization. Geneva: WHO, 2000. (WHO/V&B/00.36).

5. Chen RT, Davis RL, Sheedy KM. Safety of immunizations. In: Plotkin SA, Orenstein WA, eds. *Vaccines*, 4th ed. Philadelphia: WB Saunders Co, 2004: 1557–1581.

6. Centers for Disease Control and Prevention. Atkinson W, Hamborsky J, McIntyre L, Wolfe S, eds. *Epidemiology and prevention of vaccine-preventable diseases*, 8th ed. Washington, DC: Public Health Foundation, 2005.

7. Global Training Network on Vaccine Quality (GTN/VQ). Workshop on Establishing/Strengthening a National Immunization Safety Surveillance Programme. Cape Town, South Africa, 9–14 December 2002.

8. Grabenstein JD, Wilson JP. Are vaccines safe? Risk communication applied to vaccination. *Hosp Pharm* 1999;34(6):723–729.

9. Bayloor NW, Midthun K. Regulation and testing of vaccines. In: Plotkin SA, Orenstein WA, eds. *Vaccines*, 4th ed. Philadelphia: WB Saunders Co, 2004: 1551.

10. Greenberg DP. Pediatric experience with recombinant hepatitis B vaccines and relevant safety and immunogenicity studies [review]. *Pediatr Infect Dis J* 1993; 12(5):438–445.

11. Jefferson T, Price D, Demicheli, V, Bianco E. Unintended events following immunization with MMR: a systemic review. *Vaccine* 2003;21:3954–3960.

12. Pan American Health Organization. *Control of diphtheria, pertussis, tetanus, Haemophilus influenzae type b and hepatitis B field guide*. Scientific and Technical Publication No. 604. Washington, DC: PAHO, 2005.

13. de Oliveira LH, Struchiner CJ. Vaccine-associated paralytic poliomyelitis in Brazil, 1989–1995. *Rev Panam Salud Publica* 2000;7(4):219–224.

14. de Oliveira LH, Struchiner CJ. Vaccine-associated paralytic poliomyelitis: a retrospective cohort study of acute flaccid paralyses in Brazil. *Int J Epidemiol* 2000;29(4):757–763.

15. Centers for Disease Control and Prevention. Poliomyelitis Prevention in the United States: Introduction of a Sequential Vaccination Schedule of Inactivated Poliovirus Vaccine Followed by Oral Poliovirus Vaccine; Recommendations of the Advisory Committee on Immunization Practices (ACIP). *MMWR* 1997; 46(RR-3).

16. Centers for Disease Control and Prevention. NIP answers your questions: Polio. *What is the incidence of vaccine associated paralytic polio (VAPP) in the developing world?* http://www.cdc.gov/nip/faqs/polio-faqs.htm#OPV. Last accessed 7 June 2006.

17. World Health Organization. What to do in the event of an AEFI. http://www.who.int/immunization_safety/aefi/managing_AEFIs/en/index6.html. Last accessed 7 June 2006.

18. Burgess DC, Burgess MA, Leask J. The MMR vaccination and autism controversy in United Kingdom 1998–2005: Inevitable community outrage or a failure of risk communication? *Vaccine* 2006;24(18):3921–3928.

19. Hennekens C, Buring JE. *Epidemiology in medicine.* Mayrent SL, ed. Boston: Little, Brown, 1987.
20. Institute of Medicine. Kathleen R. Stratton, Cynthia J. Howe, eds. *Adverse events associated with childhood vaccines—evidence bearing on causality.* Washington DC: National Academy of Sciences, 1994.
21. Rothman KJ, and Greenland S, ed. *Modern epidemiology*, 2nd ed. Baltimore: Lippincott, Williams & Wilkins 1998.
22. Van Staa A, Hardon A. Injection practices in the developing world. WHO Drug Action Programme. Geneva: WHO, 1996. (WHO /DAP/96.4.).
23. World Health Organization. Department of Vaccines and Biologicals. WHO policy statement: The use of opened multi-dose vials of vaccine in subsequent immunization sessions. Geneva: WHO, 2000. (WHO/V&B/00.09).
24. World Health Organization. Department of Vaccines and Biologicals. Tool for the assessment of injection safety. Geneva: WHO, 2001. (WHO/V&B/01.30).
25. World Health Organization. Injection Practices: Rapid Assessment and Response Guide. WHO. 1 October 2002. Basic support for institutionalizing child survival II. (WHO/BCT/02.11).
26. World Health Organization. Department of Protection of the Human Environment and Department of Vaccines and Biologicals. "First, do no harm." Introducing auto-disable syringes and ensuring injection safety in immunization systems of developing countries. Geneva: WHO, 2002. (WHO/V&B/02.26).
27. World Health Organization. Department of Blood Safety and Clinical Technology. Managing an injection safety policy. The Injection Safety Policy Planner. Geneva: WHO, 2003. (WHO/BCT/03.01).
28. Heymann DL, ed. Toxic shock syndrome. In: *Control of communicable diseases manual*, 18th ed. Washington, DC: American Public Health Association, 2004: 506–507.
29. World Health Organization. Safety of injections in immunization programmes: WHO recommended policy. Geneva: WHO, 1994. (WHO/EPI/LHIS/94.1).
30. Aylward B, et al. Reducing the risk of unsafe injections in immunization programmes: financial and operational implications of various injection technologies. *Bull WHO.* 1995; 73:531–540.
31. Steinglass R, Boyd D, Grabowsky M, Laghari AG, Khan MA, Qavi A, Evans P. Safety, effectiveness and ease of use of a non-reusable syringe in a developing country immunization programme. *Bull WHO.* 1995; 73:57–63.
32. Organización Panamericana de la Salud, División de Vacunas e Inmunización. Vacunación Segura: cómo enfrentar los eventos supuestamente atribuidos a la vacunación o inmunización. Washington, DC: PAHO, 2002.
33. Ávila ML, Castillo-Solórzano C. Vacunación en la mujer embarazada. *Acta Pediátrica Costarricense* 2005;19(3).
34. Enders G. Rubella antibody titers in vaccinated and nonvaccinated women and results of vaccination during pregnancy. *Rev Infect Dis* 1985;7(suppl 1): S103–S107.
35. Centers for Disease Control and Prevention. Current trends in rubella vaccination during pregnancy—United States, 1971–1988. *MMWR* 1989; 38(17):289–293.
36. Tookey P. Pregnancy is contraindication for rubella vaccination still. *BMJ* 2001; 322 (7300):1489.

37. Centers for Disease Control and Prevention. Recommendations of the Advisory Committee on Immunization Practices (ACIP): use of vaccines and immune globulins in persons with altered immunocompetence. *MMWR* 1993;42 (RR-4):1–18.
38. Ljungman P. Vaccination in the immunocompromised host. In: Plotkin SA, Orenstein WA, eds. *Vaccines*, 4th ed. Philadelphia: WB Saunders Co, 2004: 155–167.
39. Committee on Infectious Diseases, American Academy of Pediatrics. Report of the Committee on Infectious Diseases, 22nd edition. Peter G, ed. Elk Grove, IL: American Academy of Pediatrics, 1991:48.
40. Asociación Española de Pediatría. *Manual de Vacunas en Pediatría*, 2nd ed., Latinoamericana, 2002.
41. Salisbury DM, Begg NT, eds. *Immunisation against infectious disease: the green book*. London: Department of Health.
42. Ministério da Saúde do Brasil. Recomendações por pessoas infectadas pelo HIV. Coordenação de DST e AIDS, Brasília, 2001.
43. Canadian Medical Association. (2002). *Canadian immunization guide*, 6th ed. Ottawa.
44. World Health Organization. Department of Vaccines and Biologicals. Core information for the development of immunization policy: 2002 update. (WHO/ V&B/02.28:9–11).
45. American Academy of Pediatrics. Human immunodeficiency virus infection. In: Pickering LK, ed. *Red book: 2003 report of the Committee on Infectious Diseases*, 26th ed. Elk Grove Village, IL: American Academy of Pediatrics, 2003:360–382.
46. Pan American Health Organization. Guidelines for immunizing HIV-infected persons. *EPI Newsletter* 2005;27(2):6–7.
47. Global Advisory Committee on Vaccine Safety (GACVS). Statement on Thimerosal. World Health Organization (WHO): August, 2003.
48. Institute of Medicine (IOM). *Immunization safety*. Washington, DC: National Academy of Sciences, 2005.
49. Pan American Health Organization. Update on Thimerosal and Autism. *EPI Newsletter* 2005;27(5):4.
50. Ashraf H. US expert group rejects link between MMR and autism. *Lancet*. 2001;357:1341.

INTERPRETATION OF MEASLES AND RUBELLA SEROLOGY

Andrea S. Vicari, DVM, PhD,[1] *Vance Dietz, MD, MPH, TM,*[2]
William J. Bellini, PhD,[3] *Joe Icenogle, PhD,*[4]
and Carlos Castillo-Solórzano, MD, MPH[5]

INTRODUCTION

Surveillance is an essential strategy of measles and rubella control programs. Since illnesses characterized by fever and rash are widespread and have many different causes, clinical suspicion of measles or rubella cannot confirm a case. Enzyme immunoassays (EIA) for virus-specific immunoglobulin M (IgM) are the standard laboratory method for confirming measles or rubella virus infections *(1)*. Serological results from a single serum specimen—collected at the first contact of a suspect patient with the health care system, but no later than 28 or 30 days after rash onset—are usually quite sufficient to confirm or discard a measles or rubella suspect case *(2, 3, 4)*, particularly when the disease is endemic.

After control programs were established, the incidence of measles and rubella declined significantly. The ministers of health of the countries of

---

[1] Regional Advisor on Measles, Immunization Unit, Pan American Health Organization.

[2] Chief, Global Measles Branch, Global Immunization Division, Centers for Disease Control and Prevention.

[3] Chief; Measles, Mumps, Rubella, and Herpes Viruses Branch, Division of Viral Diseases, National Center for Immunizations and Respiratory Diseases, Coordinating Center for Infectious Diseases, Centers for Disease Control and Prevention.

[4] Lead Scientist, Rubella Laboratory Team, Rubella Virus Laboratory, Measles Virus Section, National Center for Immunization and Respiratory Diseases, Centers for Disease Control and Prevention.

[5] Regional Advisor on Vaccine and Immunization, Immunization Unit, Pan American Health Organization.

the Americas resolved to eliminate measles and rubella in 1994 and in 2003, respectively. Whereas measles and rubella once were widespread in the Region, in 2004 there were only 108 confirmed measles cases and 3,103 rubella cases in the Americas. The number of confirmed cases represents less than 5% of the more than 35,000 suspect patients tested each year. Under those conditions, even though the characteristics of the EIA kits used in national laboratories are excellent, the predictive value of positive results—the likelihood that positive serological results truly identify a measles/rubella virus infection—is much lower than in places where the diseases are endemic.

In countries which have interrupted the endemic transmission of the measles or rubella viruses, IgM-positive results may present interpretation challenges for national authorities. Often, the dilemma involves establishing whether the result is positive due to an infection with an imported wild-type virus, a recent vaccination, an infection with an agent known to cross-react serologically, or some other cause. An adequate interpretation might require collecting a second convalescent sample. In any case, the interpretation must always take into account clinical and epidemiological information.

This chapter will first review the fundamentals of the immunological response to a measles/rubella virus infection and the characteristics of measles/rubella IgM EIA. Then it will discuss the interpretation of serological results for cases related to vaccination or regarded as being false-positive, and the particular use of rubella serology during pregnancy. Finally, it will present the current state of novel specimens for the serological workup of measles/rubella suspect cases.

DEVELOPMENT OF MEASLES- AND RUBELLA-SPECIFIC IMMUNOGLOBULIN M AND G FOLLOWING PRIMARY INFECTION, REEXPOSURE, AND VACCINATION

Clinical onset of measles and rubella coincides with our ability to detect specific immune responses to the measles and rubella viruses through serological methods (5, 6). Two classes of antibodies, IgM and immunoglobulin G (IgG), are routinely used in serological diagnostics. The relative serum levels of IgM and IgG antibodies in a measles-susceptible individual (a person who had not previously been exposed to measles or vaccinated with a measles-containing vaccine) in relation to the days from rash onset have been well-documented (Figure 1).

Measles- and rubella-specific IgM antibodies appear before IgG and can be detected at the time of or within days of rash onset. Whereas approximately 70% of measles cases are IgM-positive at the time of rash onset, ap-

FIGURE 1. Serological response in acute measles infection.

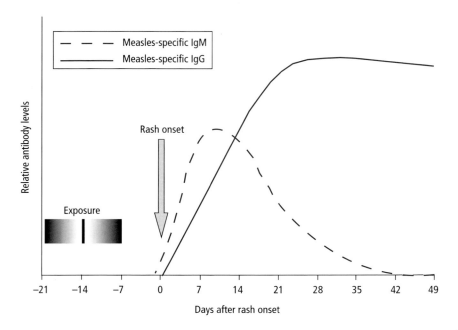

proximately 50% of rubella cases are. IgM antibodies attain peak levels approximately one week later, then gradually decline and are mostly undetectable four and six weeks after rash onset for measles and rubella, respectively. The primary difference between measles and rubella infections is that rubella-specific IgM have a slightly delayed rise and a slower decline than measles-specific IgM.

IgG antibodies appear within a week of rash onset, peak at about two weeks of rash onset, and are detectable for years after an infection. Sera of susceptible individuals will typically show a fourfold or greater increase in IgG titers in two adequately spaced specimens, the first collected during the acute phase of measles or rubella (usually with the first contact with the patient, days 0–10 after rash onset) and the second during the convalescent phase (days 14–21 after rash onset, at least 7 days after collection of first specimen).

Reexposure to measles and rubella virus in a person with pre-existing measles immunity induces a characteristic anamnestic immunologic response, with a rapid boosting of IgG levels. Serologic assays will typically not detect IgM in reexposed individuals. Primary vaccination and revaccination (of a person who responded to primary vaccination) elicits a similar pattern of serological response as seen after primary natural infection and reexposure. Although antibody levels tend to be lower after vaccination than after natural infection, these differences have no practical use in differentiating whether a rash illness is associated with a wild-type virus infection or with vaccination.

CHARACTERISTICS OF MEASLES- AND RUBELLA-SPECIFIC IGM EIA

The most commonly used methods for both IgM and IgG detection are enzyme immunoassays (EIAs), which offer the advantage of a rapid, accurate, reproducible, and efficient diagnosis (7). IgM EIA is done by using an indirect and a capture format. Changes in IgG titers—in particular the fourfold or greater rise in titers between acute and convalescent sera during acute primary infection—can be assessed with semi-quantitative IgG EIA, a plaque neutralization reduction test (PRNT), or hemagglutination inhibition (HI). Among serological methods, PRNT and HI are considered the "gold standard" for laboratory diagnosis of measles and rubella, respectively, although these methods are only carried out in specialized laboratories. By targeting neutralizing antibodies, PRNT and HI are the only methods that actually measure the property of immunity.

As discussed in the previous section, serum antibody levels vary with the natural progression of the immune response. Not surprisingly, the time between infection and serum specimen collection determines the sensitivity (the ability to correctly identify sera from infected individuals) of measles and rubella IgM EIA. Indirect and capture IgM EIA have a similar sensitivity. Commercially available measles and rubella IgM EIA generally show high specificity (the ability of discarding sera from uninfected individuals). However, some commercial EIA have showed a higher proportion of cross-reactions to agents of rash illnesses other than measles and rubella, such as dengue viruses (see section below on specificity of measles and rubella IgM EIA).

Sensitivity of Measles IgM EIA

Using an IgM capture method, Helfand and colleagues (8) looked at the measles IgM in a pool of 166 persons' seropositivity rate detected in several different settings and for whom paired serum samples were available. Among persons whose second sample was IgM-positive for measles, the first sample was IgM-positive in 77% and 100% of the persons when the first sample was collected within 3 days and between 4 and 11 days of rash onset, respectively. Among unvaccinated persons, the IgM seropositivity rate declined from 100% at four days after rash onset to 94% and

63% at four and five weeks after rash onset, respectively. The authors concluded that, when using an IgM capture EIA, a single serum specimen collected between 4 and 28 days after rash onset can be used to diagnose an acute measles virus infection.

Along with the IgM capture EIA used in the previous study, Ratnam and colleagues (9) evaluated five commercial IgM EIA, four indirect and one capture. Sera originated from 100 patients who had contracted measles during a large outbreak in Canada and who had at least a fourfold rise in measles-specific IgG titers in a paired sample. Since the date of rash onset was not available for all patients, the date of the first reported symptom (mostly fever) was used to establish the interval between illness onset and specimen collection. IgM seropositivity of the first specimen (collected on median four days after symptom onset) was between 58% and 70% for the indirect EIA; it was 77% and 80% for the capture EIA. IgM seropositivity increased with the second specimen (collected on median 18 days after symptom onset): between 92% and 96% for the indirect EIA and 97% for the capture EIA. The greatly improved rate of detection in the convalescent sera replicated previous observations (10, 11).

The previous results were only partially replicated by Tipples and colleagues (12). They contrasted three commercial IgM EIA, two capture and one indirect; 423 paired sera from measles patients reported through surveillance in Iran and confirmed by either fourfold rise in IgG or consistent IgM-positive results were tested. For the two capture EIA, IgM seropositivity was >90% on the day of rash onset and increased to >95% on day five after rash onset. For the indirect EIA, IgM seropositivity fluctuated around 85%, independently of the collection day after rash onset. Although the difference between the two capture assays and the indirect assay appeared significant, no explanation for the difference was put forward.

Sensitivity of Rubella IgM EIA

Studies on the sensitivity of rubella-specific IgM EIA gave similar outcomes to those of measles-specific IgM EIA. For instance, 72 sera from patients with primary infection, reinfection, congenital rubella, and primary vaccination were tested with 15 commercial EIA (13). Presence of rubella-specific IgM in the sera had previously been established by M-antibody capture radioimmunoassay. Sensitivities ranged from 63% to 92%. Bellini and Icenogle (14) reported 100% sensitivity at day 5 after rash onset. The influence of the time between infection and serum specimen collection on assay sensitivity was characterized in detail in a study that evaluated seven commercial rubella-specific IgM EIA (15). Four assays used an indirect format; three, a capture format. In each assay, sensitivity was tested with 174 paired sera that had been collected as part of measles/rubella surveillance in Iran from cases that had been confirmed as rubella either by IgG seroconversion, fourfold or greater rise in IgG titers, or IgM sero-conversion in convalescent serum consistently across assays. Overall, sensitivities ranged from 69% to 79%, the differences between assays not being statistically significant. Sensitivity clearly depended on when the specimen was collected: sensitivities for acute sera (all specimens were collected within 10 days of rash onset; on average, within 2 days of rash onset) ranged from 40% to 58%, whereas sensitivities for convalescent sera (all specimens collected after 10 days of rash onset; on average, 19 days of rash onset) ranged from 94% to 99%. With the exception of the day of rash onset (where sensitivity appeared higher than between days 1–14 after rash onset), >60% IgM sensitivity was first achieved with convalescent specimens (specimens collected 10 days after rash onset or later).

The strong influence of time between rash onset and specimen collection on the sensitivity of measles/rubella IgM EIA would support the need for collecting a second serum specimen whenever an early acute-phase serum specimen is IgM-negative and measles/rubella infection is suspected. However, a blanket implementation of such a principle within the surveillance context of greatly reduced or absent measles/rubella transmission (i.e., when the vast majority of thousands of specimens is negative) has important, counterintuitive implications. First, the work-load and the costs of collecting and processing a second specimen would be huge. Second, it is difficult to elicit patients' compliance once the acute phase of the illness has subsided, and the majority of cases would presumably be lost to follow-up. Third, the proportion of false-positive results could theoretically increase, augmenting the cases that are difficult to interpret (see next section). Finally, collecting a second specimen can actually reduce the timeliness of the surveillance. In a Central American country, a second specimen collected five or more days after rash onset was requested for measles and rubella diagnosis whenever a specimen collected within 72 hours of rash onset had negative test results. Over time, health center personnel began to forgo collection of a specimen at the first contact with a suspect patient, waiting instead to collect on day 5 after rash onset or later. Some cases might have been lost to follow-up before any specimen was ever collected.

As long as any suspected measles/rubella cases are the object of timely and exhaustive epidemiological follow-up (considered in the Americas as a continued requirement even after measles and rubella virus transmission is interrupted), the diminished sensitivity of an integrated measles/rubella surveillance system based on a single specimen collected at first contact with a suspect patient would not prevent achieving and maintaining measles/rubella elimination. Surveillance must remain simple to maintain the commitment of field personnel to quality.

In an outbreak, no suspect case with an established epidemiological link to a confirmed case should be discarded solely on the basis of a negative result from an early acute-phase specimen. Similarly, a second specimen is indicated for any suspect measles/rubella case who traveled to areas with measles/rubella in the 7–21 days (measles) or 12–23 days (rubella) prior to rash onset and whose early acute-phase specimen was IgM-negative.

Specificity of Measles and Rubella IgM EIA

Especially in a setting where there is little or no known transmission, measles and rubella confirmation requires a laboratory workup. However, commercial measles- and rubella-specific IgM EIA show cross-reactivity to IgM specific to other infectious agents, many of which can also cause rash illnesses difficult to distinguish clinically from measles and rubella. In measles assays, IgM cross-reactivity has been reported for patients with rubella *(12, 16)*, human parvovirus B19 infection *(12, 16, 17)*, human herpes virus 6 infection *(12)*, and dengue viruses infection (Graham Tipples, personal communication). Ratman and colleagues *(9)* also reported on sera which showed simultaneous IgM-reactivity in measles assays and in assays for either Epstein-Barr virus, cytomegalovirus, mycoplasma, or factor rheumatoid, but the authors did not give details on the actual conditions affecting the patients from whom sera originated. In rubella assays, IgM cross-reactivity has been reported for patients with measles *(15, 18)*, human parvovirus B19 infection *(15, 16)*, Epstein-Barr virus infection, mycoplasma infection, rheumatoid arthritis *(15)*, and dengue viruses infection (Graham Tipples, personal communication). In addition, reactivation of IgM responses to multiple viruses, including measles virus, rubella virus, and parvovirus B19, can occur in response to infection by one of the viruses *(16)*.

The expected rate of cross-reactions can be inferred from the observed specificity of the assays. In an evaluation of three commercial measles IgM EIA, Tipples and colleagues *(12)* compared the specificity of the assays with a nonmeasles panel comprised of 224 sera from confirmed cases of rubella (208 sera), human herpes virus 6 infection (12), and human parvovirus B19 infection (4). Overall specificities of two assays were over 98% (i.e., less than 2% of the positive results are false-positive). Although statistically smaller, the specificity of the third assay was still 95%. The rate of false-positive results varied by both the casual agent of the infection, as well as the commercial assay employed. In the evaluation of six commercial measles IgM assays, the rate of false positive results for 57 sera collected during a rubella outbreak varied from 0% to 16%, and those for 142 sera collected during a human parvovirus B19 outbreak varied from 0% to

32% *(9)*. While one assay never produced a false-positive result, two assays performed less well for both rubella and parvovirus B19 sera.

In an evaluation of seven commercial rubella IgM EIA, Tipples and colleagues *(15)* compared the specificity of the assays with nonrubella panels (between 156 and 499 sera tested in each assay) from confirmed cases of measles, human parvovirus B19 infection, Epstein-Barr virus infection, human herpes virus 6 infection, mycoplamsa infection, and rheumatoid arthritis. Five assays showed similar overall specificities (range, 94%–97%); the remaining two had a statistically significant lower specificity (86%). With the exception of sera from cases with human herpes virus 6 infection, sera from cases with the other infections resulted false-positive for rubella. As is the case with measles assays, the rate of cross-reactions varied by both the causal agent of the infection, as well as the commercial assay employed. In particular, 25% or more of the sera from three distinct set of cases gave false-positive results for rubella in an assay. Unpublished data from this study showed that of 100 sera from confirmed dengue patients, between 3 and 20 sera resulted positive (Graham Tipples, personal communication). This result is of particular significance for many countries of the Americas where dengue is endemic. Those responsible for measles/rubella surveillance should be aware of the occurrence of other rash illnesses in their geographic area of responsibility which might lead to false-positive measles/rubella IgM results.

PRACTICAL DILEMMAS IN CASE CLASSIFICATION: VACCINE-RELATED CASES AND CASES WITH SEROLOGICAL RESULTS REGARDED AS BEING FALSE-POSITIVE

When no measles case has been confirmed for years, the occurrence of an IgM-positive result generally causes great concern to national health authorities, and health officials often question the accuracy of such results. The Pan American Health Organization reviewed this issue in the Americas and established practical guidelines *(19, 20, 21)* that further expanded the conclusions from the American experience related to measles surveillance. In principle, as long as there is no evidence to the contrary, all suspect measles/rubella cases that have an IgM-positive result should be considered to be laboratory-confirmed cases. If not already under way, adequate investigation and control measures need to be initiated immediately. In a country with no known transmission, the finding of sporadic measles/rubella cases with little or no secondary transmission does not imply a resurgence of endemic measles transmission or the failure of measles/rubella elimination initiatives. The periodic finding of sporadic measles cases or small clusters of measles cases in Canada and the United States demonstrates that surveillance is sufficiently sensitive to detect imported and import-related cases from other continents (a constant threat in the Americas) and that local vaccination coverage levels are adequate to prevent epidemics. In other words, the consistent detection of sporadic measles/rubella cases that investigations link to virus importations strongly supports the maintenance of measles/rubella elimination in a country.

Nevertheless, there are two situations in which measles/rubella IgM-positive results are not associated with cases infected with wild-type measles/rubella. They must be viewed as the exception rather than the rule, and should be evaluated on a case-by-case basis. First, a patient recently vaccinated with measles- or rubella-containing vaccines who develops rash (up to 5% of individuals do after a trivalent measles-mumps-rubella [MMR] vaccination) would ideally be reported as a suspected case, and usually would have measles and/or rubella IgM-positive results. Second, as shown in the previous section, the kits for detecting measles/rubella IgM do not have 100% specificity. Some patients with rash illnesses, such as rash due to parvovirus B19 infection or dengue, may test positive for measles- or rubella-specific IgM.

Vaccine-related Cases

In addition to laboratory results, criteria to classify a case as vaccine-related should include clinical presentation, time between vaccination and illness onset, time between illness onset and sample collection, and epidemiological information. Specifically, a suspect measles/rubella case can be classified as discarded and diagnosed as a vaccine-related rash if it meets all five of the following criteria:

1. The patient had a rash illness, with or without fever, but did not have cough or other respiratory symptoms related to the rash.
2. The rash began 7–14 days after vaccination with a measles-containing vaccine.
3. The IgM-positive blood specimen was collected 8–56 days after vaccination.
4. A thorough field investigation did not identify an index case or any secondary cases.
5. Field and laboratory investigations failed to identify other causes (including the inability to detect wild-type measles/rubella virus in cultures or clinical specimens).

Obviously, the isolation or detection from a patient's specimen of a virus that has the molecular sequence of the strain contained in the vaccine single-handedly confirms a relation to the vaccine. This highlights the importance of obtaining adequate specimens for virus isolation and detection for all suspect measles/rubella cases (throat swabs collected at first contact with patients within seven days of rash onset). It is recognized that the five criteria set above will lead to confirmation of a few suspect cases whose illness actually was vaccine-related. This misclassification has to be seen as a necessary compromise to ensure the highest sensitivity and consistency of measles/rubella surveillance.

An analysis conducted in the Americas between 2003 and 2005 of suspect measles/rubella cases classified as vaccine-related (259 [0.7%] of 38,894 suspect cases reported via the Measles Elimination Surveillance System) revealed that only 38% of these cases met the criterion of rash onset 7–14 days after vaccination (22). In particular, rash onset occurred in 55% of the cases ≥15 days after vaccination (in 20% of cases ≥31 days after vaccination). Many countries in the Americas have set looser standards for the time frame in which rash develops after MMR vaccination, particularly relying on the belief that rash related to the rubella component of the MMR vaccine might occur as late as 30 days after vaccination. However, a thorough literature review and expert consultation again stressed how vaccine-related rash occurs specifically between 7 and 14 days following MMR vaccination (22). In particular, two prospective studies that included control groups found that the proportion of rash cases beyond the second week after MMR vaccination is not significantly different between vaccinated and control groups (23, 24). This finding strongly suggests that rash seen after the second week from vaccination is not related to the MMR vaccine. The published text that is often quoted to support the determination of rubella-related rash as late as 30 days after vaccination actually refers only to arthralgia (25). Cases classified as vaccine-related when rash onset actually occurs beyond 7–14 days following vaccination could originate from infection with agents other than measles and rubella virus but that also cause rash illnesses. This situation can lead to false-positive IgM results. These cases should have been followed up as described in the section that follows.

Cases with False-positive Results

While an accurate investigation often allows for confirmation of the occurrence of a vaccine-related case, evaluation of a possible false-positive IgM result is complex. From the laboratory's perspective, a conclusive answer depends on whether acute and convalescent serum specimens are available for IgG titer comparison and on whether tests for other causal agents are available and have been conducted. If acute and convalescent IgG results are not available or an alternate diagnosis cannot be confirmed with appropriate laboratory methods, a suspect case must be confirmed as measles or rubella on the basis of the IgM-positive result. With the exception of pregnant women in rubella outbreaks, false-positive results are really only an issue for sporadic measles/rubella cases.

Each IgM result regarded as being false-positive needs to be considered on a case-by-case basis, and should consider clinical presentation, vaccination history, outcome of the epidemiological investigation, and laboratory results. In the laboratory, the most critical workup is the comparison of IgG titers in paired serum specimens, with the first specimen having been collected within seven days of rash onset and the second specimen, one to two weeks thereafter. In countries with limited laboratory capabilities, this is often the only possible workup in the country (short of submitting specimens to a regional reference laboratory). Commercial measles- and rubella-specific IgG EIA are used. Algorithms for interpreting serological results for suspect measles or rubella cases with IgM-positive results regarded as being false-positive based on paired IgG titers are often useful (Figure 2). Whenever available, IgM EIA specific to agents of rash illnesses other than measles and rubella should be used to complement the comparison of measles- or rubella-specific IgG titers. In countries with the necessary laboratory capabilities, viral detection or isolation and IgG avidity assays also can be used.

In Latin America, IgM-positive sera are often retested with a second IgM EIA regarded as having better characteristics or a different format. After noting that all IgM EIA used in the Region have comparable specificity and sensitivity, Dietz and colleagues (21) concluded that this additional IgM testing should not be required nor construed as "confirmatory." However, these authors did consider it useful for reference laboratories to have a second IgM EIA in the event of a disruption in the production of the standard assay or if the quality of a particular EIA lot is in doubt. Having multiple IgM results without IgG results from paired specimens and IgM results for other agents of rash illnesses generally further confuses the interpretation of results regarded as IgM false-positive.

For the purpose of surveillance standardization, two conditions must be met before a health official may conclude that an IgM result is false-positive and discards the relative suspect measles/rubella cases. First, a thorough field investigation must have been conducted and have failed to identify any measles/rubella cases (whether an index case or secondary cases). Second, IgG titer analysis cannot be compatible with an acute measles/rubella virus infection or laboratory results must confirm a diagnosis other than measles/rubella that is compatible with the clinical presentation of the suspect patient. A suspect case should never be discarded merely on the basis of a clinical presentation that is not viewed as typical for measles/rubella.

FIGURE 2. Interpretation algorithm of serological results for suspected measles or rubella cases with IgM-positive results regarded as being false-positive based on paired IgG titers.

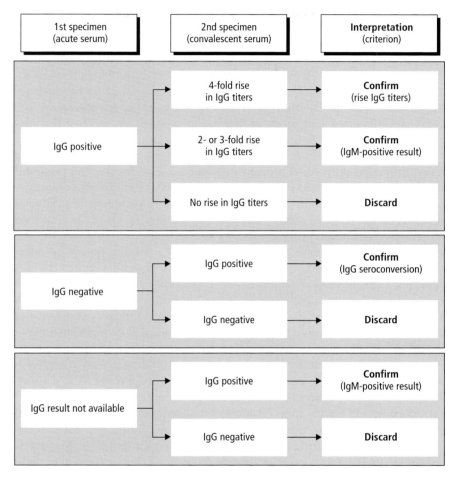

When indeterminate measles/rubella IgM or IgG results occur, serum specimens should be retested at a reference laboratory using the same assays. In the Americas, the suspect cases from which the sera originated can be discarded if three conditions are met. First, a source of infection or other suspect cases are not identified following an exhaustive epidemiological investigation. Second, measles/rubella vaccination coverage is >90% in the area where the suspect patient resides. And third, the reference laboratory reports a negative or indeterminate result.

RUBELLA DIAGNOSTICS IN PREGNANCY

Rubella infection in the first twelve weeks of pregnancy is associated with a 90% risk of congenital malformations for the newborn, also called congenital rubella syndrome (CRS). The possibility of a rubella infection always causes great anxiety to a pregnant woman and her family, and often leads to considerations of terminating the pregnancy. Consequently, laboratory results have to be evaluated, taking into account the characteristics and limitations of the applied method, as well as clinical and epidemiological information. The time between exposure and specimen collection, vaccination history, and previous laboratory results are some of the specific considerations that must be taken into account.

IgM detection should only be attempted in a pregnant woman when a recent infection with rubella virus is suspected. Specifically, the pregnant woman should have had in the previous few weeks an illness suggestive of rubella or a significant contact with someone suffering such an illness. In areas where rubella virus circulation is limited (such as in countries which have eliminated rubella or are close to that goal), IgM-positive results on serum specimens from pregnant women should always be interpreted with caution because of the low predictive positive value of the EIA assay in these settings. As mentioned in previous sections, false-positive results are known to occur because of cross-reactions with other infectious agents or autoimmune conditions. In addition, prolonged persistence of rubella-specific IgM after the usual period of six weeks from rash onset was documented in primary infection of both women and men. Rubella-specific IgM can persist for several months or even years, often at high levels (26). In these cases, rubella-specific IgG usually remain at low titers. Rubella virus reinfection has also been documented following both natural infection and vaccination. Ushida and colleagues (27) reported a CRS case in a baby born to a woman who had received one dose of rubella-containing vaccine during her teens, had rubella-specific IgG in specimens collected during two preceding pregnancies, and was exposed to wild rubella virus during the baby's pregnancy. Rubella virus reinfection poses a <5% risk of congenital damage when the mother experiences a subclinical infection; the risk for a mother with a rash illness has not been quantified (28). Although the risk of intrauterine rubella virus infection after reinfection is lower than after primary infection and occurrence of CRS in babies born to reinfected mothers is rare, the risk is not negligible. While a booster response (absence of IgM, but rapid rise and decline in IgG) would be common in case of a reinfection, a transient IgM production sometimes occurs (29). The titers of IgM produced after reinfection are usually lower and of shorter duration than after primary infection.

TABLE 1. Avidity index of sera from women who were inadvertently vaccinated with rubella vaccine and tested IgM-positive for rubella.

Days after vaccination	Number of sera	Sera by avidity index (%)		
		Low	Intermediate	High
<30	22	77	14	9
30–49	42	62	19	19
50–79	61	13	28	59
>80	45	0	11	89

Source: M. M. Siqueira, personal communication.

Consequently, susceptibility prior to exposure can only be established with a method that detects rubella-specific IgG. Guidelines from the United States Centers for Disease Control and Prevention recommend that the susceptibility status of women of childbearing age be established routinely through either verifiable proof of vaccination or an IgG-positive serologic result *(30)*. Those women who are susceptible and not pregnant would be vaccinated. Susceptible pregnant women would be vaccinated after giving birth; they should be advised to avoid contact with persons with a rash illness and should be monitored for signs of rubella during the pregnancy.

In countries with limited laboratory resources, follow-up of pregnant women suspected of being infected with rubella should at least include the collection of paired serum specimens, the first during the acute phase of the illness (within 7–10 days of rash onset) and the second during the convalescent phase of the illness (14–21 days after rash onset and at least 7 days after the first sample). It is essential that the convalescent specimen be collected regardless of the results of the first acute specimen and that the presence of both rubella-specific IgM and IgG be tested on both specimens. Unfortunately, the collection of paired specimens is not always possible, making evaluation very difficult.

An additional laboratory test that can assist in discerning the possibility of a primary rubella infection in a pregnant woman is the avidity IgG EIA. Unfortunately, as of 2006 this assay is only available at a few select laboratories. The method is based on the maturation process that IgG production undergoes with increasing time as it moves from primary exposure to a virus. Specifically, the strength of the binding between IgG and the relative antigen—called affinity—increases over time with subsequent IgG generations. While low-avidity IgG makes up the greater proportion of total humoral IgG in the initial weeks following a primary infection, high-affinity IgG increases later on. Table 1 illustrates this concept based on a study that determined avidity indexes of sera from vaccinated pregnant women who had tested IgM-positive for rubella (M. M. Siqueira, personal communication). When an affinity IgG EIA test results in a low-avidity index, recent primary infection (or vaccination) can be suspected. Within two days of rash onset, a high-avidity index could be an indication of past infection. Three or more days after rash onset, a high-avidity index is of little assistance.

ALTERNATIVE SPECIMENS FOR SEROLOGICAL DIAGNOSTIC OF MEASLES AND RUBELLA

The standard specimen for measles and rubella serology has been blood collected through phlebotomy. Upon collection, whole blood must be shipped within 24 hours to a laboratory or serum must be separated, preferably by centrifugation; storage and shipment of whole blood and serum must occur at 4°C–8°C. These collection and handling requirements pose practical challenges to a measles/rubella surveillance system. Phlebotomy is often perceived as an invasive technique by patients or parents. Environmental conditions and scarce resources in many developing countries make it a challenge to handle whole blood separation and manage to reverse cold chain conditions. Because of this, two alternative techniques for specimen collection have been developed and evaluated.

The first is based on oral fluid. The technique was first developed in the United Kingdom in the early 1990s for measles and rubella elimination programs (31, 32) and today is well-advanced for both measles and rubella diagnostics. Saliva is collected by rubbing a specially designed sponge swab around the gum margin; the swab is then put in its packaging tube and sent to a laboratory. Compared to a blood specimen, the oral fluid specimen is pain-free and simple to collect. The need for a special collection device is a potential drawback, however. In the United Kingdom, stability of the oral fluid specimens for 7 days at 20°C has been proven not to be a problem with IgM capture EIA. Specimens in the United Kingdom are shipped through regular mail service. However, specimen stability in warmer temperatures remains untested. IgM and IgG assays are available for both measles and rubella serology, and their performance has been established. Antibody levels measured in oral fluid are less precise than antibody levels measured in serum. For instance, oral fluid specimens tested with a capture EIA for measles-specific IgM showed a relative sensitivity of 71% and 90% at 0–5 days and 6–8 days after rash onset, respectively, compared to standard serum specimens (33). Because of a reduced positive predictive value in low-incidence settings, suspect measles patients with IgM-positive oral fluid specimens should be retested using a standard serum specimen. The same is true when oral fluid specimens show low levels of antibodies. As of June 2006, only one commercial assay for measles IgM was available. The ability to test other causes of rash illnesses is also limited with oral fluid specimens compared to standard serum specimens. However, nucleic acid of measles and rubella virus can be detected in oral fluid specimens with reverse transcription-polymerase chain reaction (RT-PCR). The measles virus genome was successfully sequenced in all 53 oral fluid specimens collected during an outbreak that occurred in Ethiopia *(33)*.

The second technique is based on blood drops collected on a filter paper, also referred to as "dried blood spots." As of early 2006, this technique's development was well advanced for measles diagnostics and promising for rubella diagnostics. At least three spots of venous blood collected after a finger prick are deposited on a filter paper and allowed to dry at room temperature. Once the blood drops have dried, the filter paper is put into a sealed plastic bag and, if needed, can be shipped through regular mail service. As long as the sample is kept in low humidity conditions (for instance, by adding a humidity absorbent to the sealed bag), a reverse cold chain is not required for transporting the sample to the laboratory. At the laboratory, commercially available assays can be used after the specimen has been eluted. Results show high concordance when comparing dried blood spots to standard serum specimens. Using a measles-specific IgM EIA, Riddell and colleagues *(34)* showed 100% sensitivity and 97.1% specificity of dried blood spots that had been stored at 4°C for less than six months. However, the proportion of equivocal results seemed to increase after six months of storage. In the Netherlands, comparable results were obtained on dried blood spots kept at room temperature for five months after having been stored frozen for one to two years upon collection (95% sensitivity and 96% specificity) *(35)*. In a study following vaccination, Helfand and colleagues *(36)* demonstrated good concordance of dried blood spots with standard serum samples for both measles- and rubella-specific antibodies: 98% for measles IgM, 93% for measles IgG, 94% for rubella IgM, and 93% for rubella IgG. As of November 2005, results of a study in Peru among persons with naturally acquired rubella infections are pending *(37)*. Possible limitations of laboratory testing of dried blood spots are limited blood volume for repeated or differential diagnostics and the increase in workload due to specimen elution and processing. Nevertheless, RT-PCR has been used for measles virus detection in dried blood spots *(35, 38)*.

A WHO expert panel concluded in 2004 that, once fully evaluated, the benefits of alternative sampling techniques may eventually depend on the stage of measles/rubella control in a region or country *(39)*. Specifically, experts feel that areas with endemic disease transmission could benefit most from the alternative techniques, because their easier collection and shipment requirements would simplify setting up a surveillance system. The necessity of subnational laboratories would be reduced, since specimen transportation to a national laboratory would be greatly improved. However, experts feel that areas where measles and/or rubella have been eliminated or are about to be eliminated would not substantially benefit, except where collection or shipment of standard serum specimens has proven suboptimal. Finally, supplementary collection of oral fluid specimens for virus detection and characterization should enhance the overall surveillance quality.

CONCLUSIONS

The three basic elements of a measles-rubella surveillance system are clinical suspicion, epidemiological investigation, and laboratory confirmation. Each one of these elements taken alone has specific limitations, and the strength of a surveillance system will ultimately depend on the capacity to integrate the information that each element provides. While serological assays are efficient at confirming clinical measles and rubella suspicions, serological results need to be interpreted in the context of clinical (e.g., clinical signs, timing of specimen collection) and epidemiological (e.g., contact with previous cases, travel history, occurrence of rash illnesses) information. In specific circumstances, additional specimens and testing may be indicated. Professionals with responsibility in measles and rubella control programs should be mindful of such needs.

References

1. Featherstone D, Brown D, Sanders R. Development of the Global Measles Laboratory Network. *J Infect Dis* 2003;187(suppl 1):S264–S269.
2. World Health Organization, Europe Regional Office. *Surveillance guidelines for measles and congenital rubella syndrome in the WHO European Region*. Copenhagen, Denmark: World Health Organization, Regional Office for Europe, 2003:72.
3. World Health Organization, Africa Regional Office. *Guidelines for measles surveillance*. Harare, Zimbabwe: World Health Organization, Regional Office for Africa, 2004:38.
4. Pan American Health Organization. *Measles elimination: Field guide*, 2nd ed. Washington, DC: Pan American Health Organization, 2005:97.
5. Plotkin SA, Reef S. Rubella vaccine. In: Plotkin SA, Orenstein WA, eds. *Vaccines*, 4th ed. Philadelphia: WB Saunders Co, 2004:707–743.
6. Strebel PM, Papania MJ, Halsey NA. Measles vaccine. In: Plotkin SA, Orenstein WA, eds. *Vaccines*, 4th ed. Philadelphia: WB Saunders Co, 2004;389–440.
7. Bellini WJ, Helfand RF. The challenges and strategies for laboratory diagnosis of measles in an international setting. *J Infect Dis* 2003;187(suppl 1):S283–S290.

8. Helfand RF, Heath JL, Anderson LJ, Maes EF, Guris D, Bellini WJ. Diagnosis of measles with an IgM capture EIA: the optimal timing of specimen collection after rash onset. *J Infect Dis* 1997;175:195–199.

9. Ratnam S, Tipples G, Head C, Fauvel M, Fearon M, Ward BJ. Performance of indirect immunoglobulin M (IgM) serology tests and IgM capture assays for laboratory diagnosis of measles. *J Clin Microbiol* 2000;38(1):99–104.

10. Mayo DR, Brennan T, Cormier DP, Hadler J, Lamb P. Evaluation of a commercial measles virus immunoglobulin M enzyme immunoassay. *J Clin Microbiol* 1991;29:2865–2867.

11. Ozanne G, d'Halewyn MA. Performance and reliability of the Enzygnost measles enzyme-linked immuno-sorbent assay for detection of measles virus-specific immunoglobulin M antibody during a large measles epidemic. *J Clin Microbiol* 1992;30:564–569.

12. Tipples GA, Hamkar R, Mohktari-Azad T, Gray M, Parkyn G, Head C, Ratnam S. Assessment of immunoglobulin M enzyme immunoassays for diagnosis of measles. *J Clin Microbiol* 2003;41:4790–4792.

13. Hudson P, Morgan-Capner P. Evaluation of 15 commercial enzyme immunoassays for the detection of rubella-specific IgM. *Clin Diagn Virol* 1996;5: 21–26.

14. Bellini WJ, Icenogle J. Measles and rubella virus. In: Murray P, ed., *Manual of clinical microbiology*, 8th ed. Washington, DC: American Society for Microbiology, 2003:1389–1403.

15. Tipples GA, Hamkar R, Mohktari-Azad T, Gray M, Ball J, Head C, Ratnam S. Evaluation of rubella IgM enzyme immunoassays. *J Clin Virol* 2004;30:233–238.

16. Thomas HI, Barrett E, Hesketh LM, Wynne A, Morgan-Capner P. Simultaneous IgM reactivity by EIA against more than one virus in measles, parvovirus B19 and rubella infection. *J Clin Virol* 1999;14:107–118.

17. Jenkerson SA, Beller M, Middaugh JP, Erdman DD. False positive rubeola IgM tests. *N Engl J Med* 1995;332:1103–1104.

18. Donovan SM. False-positive results of an enzyme immunoassay for rubella IgM in a case of measles. *Clin Infect Dis* 1997;24:271–272.

19. Pan American Health Organization. Measles case classification. Frequent dilemmas in the field. *EPI Newsletter* 2001;23:4–5.

20. Pan American Health Organization. Measles case classification. II. Frequent dilemmas in the field. *EPI Newsletter* 2001;23:3–4.

21. Dietz V, Rota J, Izurieta H, Carrasco P, Bellini W. The laboratory confirmation of suspected measles cases in settings of low measles transmission: conclusions from the experience in the Americas. *Bull WHO* 2004;82:852–857.

22. Pan American Health Organization. Classification of suspect measles/rubella cases as "vaccine-related": compliance with PAHO recommendations. *Immunization Newsletter* 2006;27:5.

23. Peltola H, Heinonen O. Frequency of true adverse reactions to measles-mumps-rubella vaccine. *Lancet* 1986;26:939–942.

24. Virtanen M, Peltola H, Paunio M, Heinonen OP. Day-to-day reactogenicity and the healthy vaccine effect of measles-mumps-rubella vaccination. *Pediatrics* 2000;106:E62.

25. Banatvala JE, Best JM. Rubella. In: Collier L, Balows A, Sussman M, eds. *Microbiology and microbial infections*, 9th ed. New York: Oxford University Press, 1998:571.

26. Thomas HI, Morgan-Capner P, Roberts A, Hesketh L. Persistent rubella-specific IgM reactivity in the absence of recent primary rubella and rubella reinfection. *J Med Virol* 1992;36:188–192.

27. Ushida M, Katow S, Furukawa S. Congenital rubella syndrome due to infection after maternal antibody conversion with vaccine. *Japanese J Infect Dis* 2003; 56:68–69.

28. Morgan-Capner P, Crowcroft NS, PHLS Joint Working Party of the Advisory Committees of Virology and Vaccines and Immunisation. Guidelines on the management of, and exposure to, rash illness in pregnancy (including consideration of relevant antibody screening programmes in pregnancy). *Commun Dis Public Health* 2002;5:59–71.

29. Morgan-Capner P, Hodgson J, Hambling MH, Dulake C, Coleman TJ, Boswell PA, Watkins RP, Booth J, Stern H, Best JM, et al. Detection of rubella-specific IgM in subclinical rubella reinfection in pregnancy. *Lancet* 1985;1(8423): 244–246.

30. United States Centers for Disease Control and Prevention. Control and prevention of rubella: evaluation and management of suspected outbreaks, rubella in pregnant women, and surveillance for congenital rubella syndrome. *MMWR Recomm Rep* 2001;50(RR-12):1–23.

31. Brown DW, Ramsay ME, Richards AF, Miller E. Salivary diagnosis of measles: a study of notified cases in the United Kingdom, 1991–3. *BMJ* 1994;308: 1015–1017.

32. Ramsay ME, Brugha R, Brown DW, Cohen BJ, Miller E. Salivary diagnosis of rubella: a study of notified cases in the United Kingdom, 1991–4. *Epidemiol Infect* 1998;120:315–319.

33. Nigatu W, Jin L, Cohen BJ, Nokes DJ, Etana M, Cutts FT, Brown DW. Measles virus strains circulating in Ethiopia in 1998–1999: molecular characterisation using oral fluid samples and identification of a new genotype. *J Med Virol* 2001;65:373–380.

34. Riddell MA, Leydon JA, Catton MG, Kelly HA. Detection of measles virus-specific immunoglobulin M in dried venous blood samples by using a commercial enzyme immunoassay. *J Clin Microbiol* 2002;40:5–9.

35. de Swart RL, Nur Y, Abdallah A, Kruining H, El Mubarak HS, Ibrahim SA, Van Den Hoogen B, Groen J, Osterhaus AD. Combination of reverse transcriptase PCR analysis and immunoglobulin M detection on filter paper blood samples allows diagnostic and epidemiological studies of measles. *J Clin Microbiol* 2001;39:270–273.

36. Helfand RF, Keyserling HL, Williams I, Murray A, Mei J, Moscatiello C, Icenogle J, Bellini WJ. Comparative detection of measles and rubella IgM and IgG derived from filter paper blood and serum samples. *J Med Virol* 2001;65: 751–757.

37. World Health Organization. Summary and recommendations. In: Third WHO Global Measles and Rubella Laboratory Network Meeting held in Geneva on August 25–26. Geneva: World Health Organization, 2005:5.

38. El Mubarak HS, Yuksel S, Mustafa OM, Ibrahim SA, Osterhaus AD, de Swart RL. Surveillance of measles in the Sudan using filter paper blood samples. *J Med Virol* 2004;73:624–630.

39. World Health Organization. Conclusions and recommendations. In: Meeting for the Evaluation of Alternative Sampling Methods for Measles and Rubella Case Confirmation held in Geneva on July 14. Available online: http://www. who.int/immunization_monitoring/en/ (1/11/2005). Geneva: World Health Organization, 2004:3.

PREPARING FOR THE INFLUENZA PANDEMIC

Albert Osterhaus, DVM, PhD,[1] Thais dos Santos,[2]
and Otavio Oliva, MD[3]

THE PANDEMIC THREAT

Influenza pandemics, which over time have occurred at irregular and un-predictable intervals, have been associated with substantial human morbidity, mortality, and social disruption, as well as with significant economic losses (see 1 for a review). In the 20th century, the world confronted three influenza pandemics: the 1918–1919 "Spanish flu" (A/H1N1) pandemic, the 1957 "Asian flu" (A/H2N2) pandemic, and the 1968 "Hong Kong flu" pandemic. The "Spanish flu" pandemic, by far the most devastating, caused acute illness in 25%–50% of the world's population and resulted in the death of more than 40 million people worldwide (roughly 1%–2% of the world's population); it brought an unusually high mortality among young adults. Mortality in the subsequent "Asian flu" and "Hong Kong flu" pandemics was considerably less—about 1–4 million people in each—and the highest excess mortality was among the classical risk groups, such as the elderly and people with chronic disease. Nevertheless, these two pandemics were associated with considerable morbidity, social disruption, and economic loss. Current understanding of the biology, ecology, and epidemiology of influenza A viruses indicates that we can assume that influenza pandemics will occur in the future, although at present it is impossible to predict when the next influenza pandemic will

---
[1] Department of Virology, Erasmus Medical Center, Rotterdam, The Netherlands.
[2] Technical Officer, Communicable Disease Unit, Pan American Health Organization.
[3] Regional Advisor on Viral Diseases, Communicable Disease Unit, Pan American Health Organization.

strike nor from which influenza A virus it will originate. Rapid changes in human behavior and animal ecology may even predispose the world for a more rapid spread of an influenza pandemic when it emerges. Recent advances in the development of effective antiviral drugs and vaccines using state of the art technology, as well as better surveillance in humans and animals, should provide us with more effective tools to combat a future influenza pandemic.

Wild birds are the reservoir for subtypes of influenza A viruses. To date, influenza A viruses carrying 16 antigenic subtypes of hemaglutinin (HA) and 9 antigenic subtypes of neuraminidase (NA) have been identified in wild aquatic birds and poultry (2). Since 1997, epidemiologic investigations have pointed at the direct transmission of avian influenza A viruses from poultry to humans. Moreover, the dissemination of H5N1 in wild birds in areas later observed to be affected with human cases may represent direct transmission to humans who come into contact with wild birds. In 1997, 18 persons in Hong Kong became clinically infected with an avian influenza A virus (H5N1) that had caused a highly pathogenic avian influenza (HPAI) in poultry in the same region. Six of the patients died with clinical signs of severe influenza (3, 4, 5). After culling approximately 1.5 million birds at live bird markets in Hong Kong, no other human cases of infection with this virus were identified that year. The virus appeared to lack the ability to efficiently spread from person to person.

Bird-to-human transmission of avian influenza A virus resulting in clinical disease has since been described with increasing frequency. In Southeast Asia in 1999, infection with avian influenza A virus H9N2 and H5N1 caused a limited number of clinical human infections, and at least one person died (6, 7). During a large HPAI outbreak among poultry in the Netherlands in 2003, in which more than 30 million chickens had to be culled, the causative HPAI virus (H7N7) also was identified in 86 humans who had handled affected poultry and in three of their family members (8, 9). The virus was closely related to low pathogenic avian influenza (LPAI) viruses identified in wild ducks prior to the outbreak (8). The infected humans suffered from conjunctivitis and/or influenza-like illness, but the infection also resulted in fatal pneumonia with acute respiratory distress syndrome in one person (8, 9). Subsequently, human infections with avian influenza A viruses (H7N2 and H7N3) occurred in the United States in 2003 and in Canada in 2004, resulting in one and two clinical cases, respectively (6, 10, 11). Since December 2003, a rapidly increasing number of human infections with an avian influenza A virus (H5N1) have been identified in Southeast Asia, where direct or indirect contact with infected poultry and their excreta were the most likely source of infection in most, if not all, the cases. In Azerbaijan, Cambodia, China, Djibouti, Egypt, Indonesia, Iraq, Thailand, Turkey, and Vietnam, more than 200 human cases of infection with this virus have been identified, with a case fatality rate higher than 50% (for an update, visit www.who.int/csr/disease/avian_ influenza). Most of these infections were associated with respiratory disease, although diarrhea and neurological symptoms without severe respiratory disease also have been described in one or two patients (12).

The pathogenicity of this H5N1 virus for different mammalian species upon experimental infection seems to have increased gradually over time (13). Fatal infections in tigers and leopards fed with chicken carcasses have been reported; probable animal-to-animal transmission also has occurred in tigers (14, 15). Experimental infection of domestic cats resulted in systemic spread of the virus, and animal-to-animal spread has been observed as well (16, 17). In the first four months of 2006, the influenza A virus (H5N1) spread westward through Asia, probably with migratory birds, and reached the European Union. Wild and/or domestic birds became infected in 54 countries (for an update, visit http://www.oie.int/ downld/AVIAN%20INFLUENZA/A_AI-Asia.htm). In Turkey, where the virus caused extensive outbreaks of HPAI in poultry, 12 people became clinically infected after direct or indirect contacts with affected poultry; four died.

The crucial question today is whether these ongoing zoonotic events of the past decade increase the risk of the emergence of an influenza pandemic in humans. Until 1997, it was generally believed that the main risk involved the simultaneous infection of a mammalian species, such as the pig, with a human and an avian influenza A virus. This could then result in the emergence of a reassortant virus that could efficiently spread among humans in the virtual absence of pre-existing specific immunity in the human population at large. In fact, the "Asian flu" and "Hong Kong flu" pandemics were caused by viruses that were reassortants between avian and mammalian influenza A viruses. Direct infection of humans by avian influenza A viruses, as has been seen extensively since 1997, would create the possibility that such reassortant viruses could directly emerge in humans, if such infections occurred during episodes of epidemic influenza in humans.

A second scenario that could lead to the emergence of a pandemic influenza virus would be if an avian influenza A virus infected humans and gradually adapted to humans by sequential mutation, which could then open the door to efficient human-to-human transmission. The "Spanish flu" pandemic virus was probably not a result of a reassortment event; the virus probably adapted to humans by sequential mutation, although it is unknown whether other mammalian species were involved (18, 19). It is currently difficult to predict whether the ongoing influenza A virus (H5N1) infections in humans in Eurasia will lead to the next influenza pandemic. However, even if they do not, it is important to consider the urgency of having in place early warning systems and pandemic preparedness plans to cope with such an event.

Several countries have stepped up their efforts by creating national preparedness committees that have drafted and put in place national plans. Nonetheless, much work remains to be done for countries to be adequately prepared.

VACCINES FOR PANDEMIC INFLUENZA: WHERE DO THEY STAND?

In 1999, the World Health Organization (WHO) developed the first comprehensive staged plan for responding to a pandemic influenza threat. In the past, work primarily had been based on human virological surveillance activities for epidemic influenza, in which a national influenza center and WHO collaborating centers have participated actively for more than half a century. The program has been updated continuously, and recently led to the development of the WHO Global Agenda on Influenza (www.who.int/influenza), whose mission was expanded from surveillance to pandemic preparedness, assessment of the impact of influenza, and increased influenza vaccine usage. The cornerstone of pandemic influenza preparedness is the ability to rapidly produce and distribute a specific pandemic vaccine. Given the lead time required to develop and produce such a vaccine, it will certainly not be available for distribution during the first six months of a pandemic outbreak. Therefore, to bridge the gap between the onset of the outbreak and the initial pandemic vaccine distribution, stockpiles of antiviral drugs may be an important adjunct in the efforts to reduce the spread of the virus, as well as morbidity and mortality in this period. Mainly due to pre-existing or rapidly developing antiviral resistance, the oldest anti-influenza drugs—the adamantanes—will probably be of little use. New generation anti-influenza drugs—the neuraminidase inhibitors (NIs)—are, therefore, probably the drugs of choice. Because these drugs may develop antiviral resistance when used extensively, the use of combinations of different groups of antiviral drugs may be advisable (20). Furthermore, it should be kept in mind that the current global production capacity for the NIs will only allow production to cover therapeutic use for 1%–2% of the world's population. License agreement between the current NI producing companies and other companies elsewhere in the world may help lessen supply problems.

Production, distribution capacity, and efficacy also are key issues of pandemic influenza vaccines. Current epidemic or inter-pandemic influenza vaccines are predominantly inactivated subunit—split—or whole-virus vaccines, although recently cold-adapted live attenuated vaccines (CAIV-T) also have been introduced (21). All these vaccines are still produced with embryonated chicken eggs as the production substrate, which greatly limits the flexibility of production capacity. Therefore, the recent advent of cell-culture systems as a substrate, using continuous cell lines like MDCK and Vero cells, is considered to be a great improvement *(22, 23)*. This advance will create a continuous availability of production capacity with great possibilities for further improvement and optimization of production processes. Several commercial companies are now focusing on these technologies, and the first vaccines produced by cell culture may soon be available.

The rapid generation of vaccine seed strains is another area that may help reduce lead time. Today, seed viruses are produced by WHO collaborating centers when WHO recommends an antigenically new epidemic influenza virus strain for inclusion in the inter-pandemic vaccine. Classically, these vaccine seed strains are produced by double infection of embryonated chicken eggs, using the recommended virus strain and the laboratory strain PR8 (which grows to high titers in these eggs), in order to produce a high growth reassortment. The use of reverse genetics for this purpose offers several advantages over the classical reassortment approach: it is a more rational and direct approach, it saves time, and it solves the problem of the possible presence of advantageous viruses in the epidemic virus isolate that could eventually contaminate the vaccine seed strain. Finally, it offers the opportunity to modify the HA at the plasmid stage to remove pathogenic traits, like a basic cleavage site. The latter may be performed by replacing the basic cleavage site from a HPAI virus with that of a LPAI virus. A high-throughput virus backbone may be adjusted to a cell line validated for vaccine production like MDCK or Vero cells under quality-controlled conditions *(24, 25)*. Reverse genetics also may play a role in the generation of increased virus or HA yields in such new cell substrates.

The process of generating vaccine seed strains for pandemic vaccines by reassortment or reverse genetics may be bypassed by directly using LPAI ancestor or related viruses from wild bird surveillance activities *(26, 27)*. Alternatively, using reverse genetics, the whole HA from such a related LPAI virus may be used to directly construct a LPAI seed strain using a high throughput virus backbone *(27)*. Therefore, ongoing surveillance programs for wild birds, which are important as an early warning system for the emergence of HPAI, may also lead to the generation of repertoires of LPAI viruses related to possible future pandemic human influenza viruses. Viruses from such repositories can then be used directly for the rapid development of vaccine seed strains. A prerequisite for this approach is that ongoing and extended adequate analyses of antigenic properties of such LPAI viruses from both Eurasian and American lineages be carried out in such a way that they eventually allow the selection of prototype vaccine seed strains with the matching antigenic properties. This may be accomplished using the principles of recently published antigenic cartography studies based on multidimensional scaling algorithms (28).

The inactivated, inter-pandemic influenza vaccines currently in use are based predominantly on the principle of inducing virus-neutralizing (and HA-inhibiting) antibodies directed against the HA of the virus. For example, the use of vaccines consisting of only HA, produced as recombinant protein expressed by highly efficient alternative production systems like baculovirus systems, is also being considered for epidemic and pandemic influenza vaccines (29). Little attention is being paid to the contributory role of the NA of the virus in this regard. Given that only 9 NA subtypes have been identified, versus 16 HA subtypes of influenza A viruses, and that the NA is probably also less subjected to antigenic drift than the HA, efforts should be directed to better understand the potential of NA as an immunogen. This can also induce virus-neutralizing antibodies. When repositories of potential pandemic virus seed strains are being prepared, the potential of the NA to induce more broadly protective immune responses deserves further attention. A third influenza A virus protein that may elicit protective antibody responses is the M2 protein. M2 is minimally immunogenic upon natural infection and conventional vaccination, which may explain its relative conservation among human influenza A viruses. However, it has been documented that the external domain of this protein (M2e), when linked to an appropriate carrier such as hepatitis B viral core particles, becomes highly immunogenic, inducing antibodies that may protect mice against lethal influenza virus challenge (30). Although these results have not been confirmed by some groups of investigators, whose studies only showed weak protection-mediated antibody-dependent NK cell activity (31), other investigators have shown exacerbated disease in pigs after challenge with this approach (32). Additional studies are needed, because they may lead to more broadly protective vaccines that could protect against emerging pandemic influenza viruses.

The correlates of protection against influenza virus infection or disease are still poorly understood. In addition to virus-neutralizing antibodies directed against the HA, the NA, or M2e, it is not known to what extent cell-mediated immunity plays a protective role. Cell-mediated immunity may be directed to proteins other than the surface glycoproteins, such as the more conserved regions of the internal proteins, thus providing broad cross-reactive immunity between different virus subtypes. So far, limited work has been done in this area that may eventually contribute to the development of broader cross-reactive vaccines. In principle, the new generation of live attenuated CAIV may be expected to induce cytotoxic T cell (CTL) mediated immunity similar to natural infection. However, CAIV-T vaccines are based on the so-called 2–6 reverse genetics system, in which only the HA and the NA are expressed on a high-throughput backbone. Thus, CTL responses generated to the internal proteins of the CAIV may not cross-react with those of emerging pandemic viruses. Using classical non-adjuvanted formulations of inactivated vaccines for prototype pandemic vaccines in preclinical studies, and recently also in clinical trials, it was shown that multiple injections, even with high antigen concentrations, failed to induce virus-neutralizing antibody levels that were protective in animal models or that may be protective in humans *(33, 34)*. Consequently, human trials with adjuvanted prototype pandemic vaccines should be carried out immediately to demonstrate their efficacy with regard to their ability to induce adequate levels of virus-neutralizing antibody, as well as to determine their safety. The limited numbers of human trials carried out so far with alum or MF59 adjuvanted prototype vaccines have shown that at least two injections should be given with relatively high concentrations of HA. Both for antigen sparing strategies and for the reduction of the number of vaccine injections needed to induce protective immunity, additional human trials with other adjuvants should be carried out as soon as possible (Table 1).

GLOBAL INFLUENZA-VACCINE SUPPLY

The development, production, and worldwide distribution of pandemic influenza vaccines pose major problems. The first priority for producing

TABLE 1. Main opportunities for improving pandemic influenza vaccines, current scenarios, and likely improvements in the future.

Opportunities	Current scenario	Future improvements
Strain selection	Human surveillance	• Antigenic mapping techniques • Bird surveillance (repositories)
Seed-strain production	Classical reassortment	• Reverse genetics
Production substrate	Embryonated hen's eggs	• Continuous cell lines • Recombinant HA (and other) proteins (e.g., baculovirus system)
Vaccination targets based on correlates of protection	HA proteins	• N proteins • M2 proteins • Cell-mediated immunity • Mucosal immunity
Adjuvants for inactivated vaccines	Unadjuvanted (exception: MF59)	• Aluminium salts • MF59 • Virosomes • Iscoms • Others

a pandemic vaccine is the prompt development of vaccine seed strains, using state-of-the-art technology with available virus strains. Issues ranging from intellectual property rights, to novel technology such as reverse genetics, to virus strains, to production technology using continuous cell lines, for example, should be solved in the inter-pandemic period. It is not absolutely clear at this juncture which inactivated-vaccine formulation should be used, nor with which adjuvant, antigen concentration, or number of injections to provide safe and effective protection against a newly emerging pandemic influenza virus. As already said, human vaccine trials to demonstrate safety and efficacy of prototype pandemic vaccines should be carried out as soon as possible to solve these problems. Inter-pandemic influenza vaccines are unique from a licensing point of view, since the licensing process includes a procedure for rapid annual updates of vaccine strains (24). In the event of an influenza pandemic, regulatory authorities also should anticipate a rapid licensing process of new vaccines. Moreover, national agencies should make arrangements to compensate vaccine producers in case liability claims are filed against them.

Vaccine-production capacity that relies on currently available technology using embryonated chicken eggs definitely will not be able to produce sufficient pandemic vaccines for the world's needs (35). Although the use of inter-pandemic influenza vaccine is on the rise, especially in less developed countries, 60%–70% of the world's influenza vaccine is currently being produced in Europe. The best pandemic preparedness in terms of vaccine production capacity and distribution is an increased use of inter-pandemic vaccine. For this reason, Canada has considerably increased its domestic inter-pandemic vaccine production and use (36) and the European Scientific Working Group on Influenza (ESWI) has advocated an increase of the annual epidemic vaccination coverage to one-third of the population in Europe (www.eswi.org). It also is important to state here that preparedness planning for an influenza pandemic is not a public health priority for many developing countries; consequently, inter-pandemic vaccination coverage in these countries is low. Equitable distribution of pandemic influenza vaccine throughout the world is, therefore, a key issue that also should be addressed urgently (Box 1).

STRATEGIC PLAN CONSIDERATIONS: ESTABLISHING INFLUENZA TASK FORCES

Preparedness plans for an influenza pandemic should be developed, continuously updated, and tested by all national agencies responsible for public health, following recommendations included in WHO's Global Agenda on Influenza (www.who.int/influenza). To ensure that every country in

> **BOX 1.** Key issues to be resolved in the inter-pandemic phase if vaccines are to be quickly produced and distributed worldwide during a pandemic.
>
> - Vaccine seed virus strains must be developed in a timely way, on the basis of surveillance data and using state-of-the-art-technology.
> - Safe and effective prototype pandemic influenza vaccines should be identified in human clinical trials, with special attention given to adjuvants for inactivated vaccines that allow the induction of protective immunity, preferably with one injection and with minimal antigen contents of the vaccines.
> - Fast registration and licensing procedures of candidate pandemic influenza vaccines must be put in place by regulatory authorities, allowing for a rapid global use of a pandemic vaccine.
> - Problems with intellectual property rights associated with novel vaccine development and production technology must be resolved.
> - Compensation for liability claims must be set up for vaccine developers.
> - Use of inter-pandemic influenza vaccine should be increased to levels that would allow for the production and global distribution of pandemic influenza vaccines.
> - Problems related to the equitable and timely global distribution of pandemic influenza vaccines must be resolved.

the world is fully prepared for the next influenza pandemic, efforts in this area by the responsible national agencies should be stepped up drastically. Because influenza pandemics, like most virus infections that threaten human health, originate in animal reservoirs, a pandemic outbreak response will require the involvement of many disciplines. To fully understand the global threat posed by avian influenza, well-coordinated investigations of influenza viruses in wild birds and poultry populations should be an essential part of the global pandemic preparedness agenda *(37)*.

The spread of severe acute respiratory syndrome (SARS) is yet another recent, global public health threat by a virus infection that spilled over from an animal reservoir. SARS originated in Asia and rapidly spread to many countries in the world, infecting about 8,000 people, of whom about 800 died. WHO's role in the response to this outbreak was exemplary. The Organization constituted expert teams to rapidly respond to this emerging global health threat, one of which was the WHO SARS etiology team. That team consisted of laboratories in the region where the outbreak originated and laboratories with specific expertise in the area of emerging infectious diseases in other places of the world. This coordinated response resulted in the rapid identification and characterization of the etiological agent— SARS coronavirus (SARS CoV)—and the development of effective intervention strategies in just a couple of weeks *(38–41)*. Although the epidemiological features of influenza viruses are quite different from those of the

SARS-CoV, this experience showed that global interdisciplinary collaboration under the leadership of a UN organization such as WHO should definitely be considered key to combat an emerging influenza pandemic.

On September 30, 2005, UN Secretary General Kofi Anan announced the appointment of a United Nations system coordinator for pandemic influenza. This new appointment is designed to coordinate relevant agencies within the UN system, both to guide the centralized response to such an event and to provide support to Member States in this effort. Priority activities that are being promoted include early viral detection of influenza viruses in wild and domestic birds and in other animal species as a first line of defense against pandemic influenza. Surveillance in humans should continue to rely on WHO's influenza surveillance network, but should also enhance such surveillance so as to comply with the more sensitive requirements of the Organization's newly adopted International Health Regulations (IHR-2005). The initiative also will provide support to Member States in their efforts to develop national influenza pandemic preparedness plans, especially in developing countries.

Although the containment of a pandemic has never been attempted before, encouraging models have recently emerged. Two groups have demonstrated that with adequate early detection of human-to-human transmission it may be possible to halt an influenza pandemic in its earliest stages through targeted mass prophylactic use of antiviral drugs and the adoption of non-pharmaceutical interventions *(42)*. In order to make such an approach viable, early detection and rapid outbreak response systems must be in place in every country in accordance with WHO guidelines and in coordination with other specialized UN agencies, such as the World Organization for Animal Health (OIE) and the Food and Agriculture Organization (FAO).

INFLUENZA PREPAREDNESS IN THE AMERICAS

During the Presidential Summit of the Americas in Mar del Plata, Argentina, in November 2005, the Region's countries committed themselves, with the support of the Pan American Health Organization (PAHO), to completing their national plans to face the potential threat posed by the current outbreak of influenza H5N1 (see Table 2 for the status of these preparedness plans). Before this commitment had been made, PAHO had established an interprogrammatic and multidisciplinary task force on epidemic alert and response (the EAR Task Force) to meet the increased demand for technical cooperation necessitated by the emergence of an influenza strain with pandemic potential. The EAR Task Force has been charged with advising, coordinating, and monitoring all PAHO activities related to the planning and implementation of influenza pandemic pre-

TABLE 2. Status of national influenza pandemic preparedness plans, Region of the Americas, as of May 16, 2006.

Country	Ongoing preparedness activities	Draft plan received by PAHO	Plan published or available on the Internet	Plan endorsed by country authorities
Antigua and Barbuda	YES	NO	NO	NO
Argentina	YES	YES	YES	YES
Bahamas	YES	NO	NO	NO
Barbados	YES	YES	NO	NO
Belize	YES	YES	NO	NO
Bolivia	YES	YES	YES	YES
Brazil	YES	YES	YES	YES
Canada	YES	YES	YES	YES
Chile	YES	YES	YES	YES
Colombia	YES	YES	YES	YES
Costa Rica	YES	YES	NO	YES
Cuba	YES	YES	NO	YES
Dominica	YES	YES	NO	NO
Dominican Republic	YES	YES	NO	NO
Ecuador	YES	YES	YES	YES
El Salvador	YES	YES	NO	NO
Grenada	YES	NO	NO	NO
Guatemala	YES	YES	NO	NO
Guyana	YES	YES	NO	NO
Haiti	YES	NO	NO	NO
Honduras	YES	YES	NO	NO
Jamaica	YES	NO	NO	NO
Mexico	YES	YES	YES	YES
Nicaragua	YES	YES	NO	YES
Panama	YES	YES	YES	YES
Paraguay	YES	YES	NO	NO
Peru	YES	YES	YES	YES
Puerto Rico	YES	YES	NO	NO
Saint Kitts and Nevis	YES	NO	NO	NO
Saint Lucia	YES	NO	NO	NO
Saint Vincent and the Grenadines	YES	YES	NO	NO
Suriname	YES	YES	NO	NO
Trinidad and Tobago	YES	YES	NO	NO
United States of America	YES	YES	YES	YES
Uruguay	YES	YES	YES	YES
Venezuela	YES	YES	YES	NO

Source: Immunization Unit, Pan American Health Organization.

paredness and response. All EAR Task Force activities are framed under the new mandates set forth in WHO's International Health Regulations 2005 (IHR-2005), which stipulate that countries should develop, strengthen, and maintain core capacities to detect, assess, and intervene rapidly to control events of international public health importance related to risk or disease. The task force's interprogrammatic nature responds to the complex process involved in the implementation and influenza pandemic planning contemplated in IHR-2005. This work also requires that a variety of sectors, including the private sector, participate in highly coordinated efforts.

Under EAR Task Force's interprogrammatic framework, technical cooperation in influenza preparedness has included providing support to Member States to develop their national influenza pandemic preparedness plans (NIPPPs). PAHO has distributed multi-language guidelines to assist in the effort. Subregional workshops using modeling software have been conducted to estimate the potential impact of a pandemic based on multiple scenarios. The results of the modeling exercises have helped ensure that the countries' plans are flexible and can respond to many contingencies, including a worst-case scenario where there are neither available vaccines nor antiviral medications. This planning also highlights the need for the NIPPPs to prioritize interventions and address other important issues, such as access to health care.

PAHO has developed an assessment tool, based on WHO's checklist for influenza preparedness (http://www.who.int/csr/resources/publications/ influenza/FluCheck6web.pdf), to assess national plans. Assessment exercises with multidisciplinary country delegations allow for comprehensive self-assessments to be made of national influenza pandemic preparedness plans and for the exchange of ideas and strategies between countries. Important lessons learned have highlighted the need to address chain-of-command and coordination issues that may be encountered during a pandemic or during the pandemic alert period. In the Americas, countries also have conducted simulation exercises. Based on them, action plans should be developed aimed at filling the gaps identified by the self-assessments and by the simulations. Further multisectoral collaboration in the refinement of such plans will be needed.

PAHO also supports its Member States in operationalizing national influenza preparedness plans at the local level, to ensure an effective response to a pandemic. To this end, pilot interventions have been carried out in selected countries as a way to harmonize the local implementation of national plans, thus ensuring that communities at the front line of a possible pandemic will be prepared.

References

1. Potter CW. Chronicles of influenza pandemics. In: Nicholson KG, Webster RG, Hay AJ, eds. *Textbook of influenza*. Malden, MA: Blackwell Publishing, 1998: 3–18.
2. Fouchier RA, Munster V, Wallensten A, Bestebroer TM, Herfst S, Smith D, Rimmelzwaan GF, Olsen B, Osterhaus AD. Characterization of a novel in-

fluenza A virus hemagglutinin subtype (H16) obtained from black-headed gulls. *J Viral* 2005;79(5):2814–2822.

3. de Jong JC, Claas EC, Osterhaus AD, Webster RG, Lim WL. A pandemic warning? *Nature* 1997;389(6651):554.

4. Claas EC, Osterhaus AD, van Beek R, De Jong JC, Rimmelzwaan GF, Senne DA, Krauss S, Shortridge KF, Webster RG. Human influenza A H5N1 virus related to a highly pathogenic avian influenza virus. *Lancet.* 1998 Feb 14;351 (9101):472–477. Erratum in: *Lancet* 1998;351(9111):1292.

5. Subbarao K, Klimov A, Katz J, Regnery H, Lim W, Hall H, Perdue M, Swayne D, Bender C, Huang J, Hemphill M, Rowe T, Shaw M, Xu X, Fukuda K, Cox N. Characterization of an avian influenza A (H5N1) virus isolated from a child with a fatal respiratory illness. *Science* 1998;279(5349):393–396.

6. Lin YP, Shaw M, Gregory V, Cameron K, Lim W, Klimov A, Subbarao K, Guan Y, Krauss S, Shortridge K, Webster R, Cox N, Hay A. Avian-to-human transmission of H9N2 subtype influenza A viruses: relationship between H9N2 and H5N1 human isolates. *Proc Natl Acad Sci U S A* 2000;97(17):9654–9658.

7. Peiris M, Yuen KY, Leung CW, Chan KH, Ip PL, Lai RW, Orr WK, Shortridge KF. Human infection with influenza H9N2. *Lancet* 1999;354(9182):916–917.

8. Fouchier RA, Schneeberger PM, Rozendaal FW, Broekman JM, Kemink SA, Munster V, Kuiken T, Rimmelzwaan GF, Schutten M, Van Doornum GJ, Koch G, Bosman A, Koopmans M, Osterhaus AD. Avian influenza A virus (H7N7) associated with human conjunctivitis and a fatal case of acute respiratory distress syndrome. *Proc Natl Acad Sci U S A* 2004;101(5):1356–1361.

9. Koopmans M, Wilbrink B, Conyn M, Natrop G, van der Nat H, Vennema H, Meijer A, van Steenbergen J, Fouchier R, Osterhaus A, Bosman A. Transmission of H7N7 avian influenza A virus to human beings during a large outbreak in commercial poultry farms in the Netherlands. *Lancet* 2004;363(9409): 587–593.

10. Olofsson S, Kumlin U, Dimock K, Arnberg N. Avian influenza and sialic acid receptors: more than meets the eye? *Lancet Infect Dis* 2005;5(3):184–188.

11. Hirst M, Astell CR, Griffith M, Coughlin SM, Moksa M, Zeng T, et al. Novel avian influenza H7N3 strain outbreak, British Columbia. *Emerg Infect Dis* 2004;10(12):2192–2195.

12. de Jong MD, Bach VC, Phan TQ, Vo MH, Tran TT, Nguyen BH, Beld M, Le TP, Truong HK, Nguyen VV, Tran TH, Do QH, Farrar J. *N Engl J Med* 2005;352(7): 686–691.

13. Maines TR, Lu XH, Erb SM, Edwards L, Guarner J, Greer PW, Nguyen DC, Szretter KJ, Chen LM, Thawatsupha P, Chittaganpitch M, Waicharoen S, Nguyen DT, Nguyen T, Nguyen HH, Kim JH, Hoang LT, Kang C, Phuong LS, Lim W, Zaki S, Donis RO, Cox NJ, Katz JM, Tumpey TM. Avian influenza (H5N1) viruses isolated from humans in Asia in 2004 exhibit increased virulence in mammals. *J Virol* 2005;79(18):11788–11800.

14. Keawcharoen J, Oraveerakul K, Kuiken T, Fouchier RA, Amonsin A, Payungporn S, Noppornpanth S, Wattanodorn S, Theambooniers A, Tantilertcharoen R, Pattanarangsan R, Arya N, Ratanakorn P, Osterhaus DM, Poovorawan Y. Avian influenza H5N1 in tigers and leopards. *Emerg Infect Dis* 2004;10(12): 2189–2191.

15. Thanawongnuwech R, Amonsin A, Tantilertcharoen R, Damrongwatanapokin S, Theamboonlers A, Payungporn S, Nanthapornphiphat K, Ratanamungk-

lanon S, Tunak E, Songserm T, Vivatthanavanich V, Lekdumrongsak T, Kes-
dangsakonwut S, Tunhikorn S, Poovorawan Y. Probable tiger-to-tiger transmission of avian influenza H5N1. *Emerg Infect Dis* 2005;11(5):699–701. Erratum
in: *Emerg Infect Dis* 2005;11(6):976.

16. Kuiken T, Rimmelzwaan G, van Riel D, van Amerongen G, Baars M, Fouchier
R, Osterhaus A. Avian H5N1 influenza in cats. *Science* 2004;306(5694):241.
Epub 2004 Sep 2.

17. Rimmelzwaan GF, van Riel D, Baars M, Bestebroer TM, van Amerongen G,
Fouchier RA, Osterhaus AD, Kuiken T. Influenza A virus (H5N1) infection in
cats causes systemic disease with potential novel routes of virus spread within
and between hosts. *Am J Pathol* 2006;168(1):176–183.

18. Taubenberger JK, Reid AH, Krafft AE, Bijwaard KE, Fanning TG. Initial genetic characterization of the 1918 "Spanish" influenza virus. *Science* 1997;275
(5307):1793–1796.

19. Tumpey TM, Basler CF, Aguilar PV, Zeng H, Solorzano A, Swayne DE, et al.
Characterization of the reconstructed 1918 Spanish influenza pandemic virus.
Science 2005;310(5745):77–80.

20. de Jong MD, Tran TT, Truong HK, Vo MH, Smith GJ, Nguyen VC, et al. Os-
eltamivir resistance during treatment of influenza A (H5N1) infection. *N Engl
J Med* 2005;353(25):2667–2672.

21. Belshe RB. Current status of live attenuated influenza virus vaccine in the US.
Virus Res. 2004;103(1–2):177–185.

22. Brands R, Visser J, Medema J, Palache AM, van Scharrenburg GJ. Influvac: a
safe Madin Darby Canine Kidney (MDCK) cell culture-based influenza vaccine. *Dev Biol Stand* 1999;98:93–100; discussion 111.

23. Oxford JS, Manuguerra C, Kistner O, Linde A, Kunze M, Lange W, et al. A
new European perspective of influenza pandemic planning with a particular
focus on the role of mammalian cell culture vaccines. *Vaccine* 2005;23(46–47):
5440–5449.

24. Nicolson C, Major D, Wood JM, Robertson JS.Generation of influenza vaccine
viruses on Vero cells by reverse genetics: an H5N1 candidate vaccine strain
produced under a quality system. *Vaccine* 2005;23(22):2943–2952.

25. Webby RJ, Perez DR, Coleman JS, Guan Y, Knight JH, Govorkova EA,
McClain-Moss LR, Peiris JS, Rehg JE, Tuomanen EI, Webster RG. Responsiveness to a pandemic alert: use of reverse genetics for rapid development of influenza vaccines. *Lancet* 2004;363(9415):1099–1103.

26. Munster VJ, Wallensten A, Baas C, Rimmelzwaan GF, Schutten M, Olsen B,
Osterhaus AD, Fouchier RA. Mallards and highly pathogenic avian influenza
ancestral viruses, northern Europe. *Emerg Infect Dis* 2005;11(10):1545–1551.

27. de Wit E, Munster VJ, Spronken MI, Bestebroer TM, Baas C, Beyer WE, Rimmelzwaan GF, Osterhaus AD, Fouchier RA. Protection of mice against lethal
infection with highly pathogenic H7N7 influenza A virus by using a recombinant low-pathogenicity vaccine strain. *J Virol* 2005;79(19):12401–12407.

28. Smith DJ, Lapedes AS, de Jong JC, Bestebroer TM, Rimmelzwaan GF, Osterhaus AD, Fouchier RA. Mapping the antigenic and genetic evolution of influenza virus. *Science* 2004;305(5682):371–376. Epub 2004 Jun 24.

29. Fiers W, De Filette M, Birkett A, Neirynck S, Min Jou W. A "universal" human
influenza A vaccine. *Virus Res* 2004;103(1–2):173–176. Review.

30. Jegerlehner A, Schmitz N, Storni T, Bachmann MF. Influenza A vaccine based on the extracellular domain of M2: weak protection mediated via antibody-dependent NK cell activity. *J Immunol* 2004;172(9):5598–5605.

31. Heinen PP, Rijsewijk FA, de Boer-Luijtze EA, Bianchi AT. Vaccination of pigs with a DNA construct expressing an influenza virus M2-nucleoprotein fusion protein exacerbates disease after challenge with influenza A virus. *J Gen Virol* 2002;83(Pt 8):1851–1859.

32. Rimmelzwaan GF, Claas EC, van Amerongen G, de Jong JC, Osterhaus AD. ISCOM vaccine induced protection against a lethal challenge with a human H5N1 influenza virus. *Vaccine* 1999;17(11–12):1355–1358.

33. Stephenson I, Bugarini R, Nicholson KG, Podda A, Wood JM, Zambon MC, Katz JM. Cross-reactivity to highly pathogenic avian influenza H5N1 viruses after vaccination with nonadjuvanted and MF59-adjuvanted influenza A/Duck/Singapore/97 (H5N3) vaccine: a potential priming strategy. *J Infect Dis* 2005;191(8):1210–1215. Epub 2005 Mar 14.

34. Fedson DS. Vaccination for pandemic influenza: a six point agenda for inter-pandemic years. *Pediatr Infect Dis J* 2004;23(1 suppl):S74–S77.

35. Tam T, Sciberras J, Mullington B, King A. Fortune favours the prepared mind: a national perspective on pandemic preparedness. *Can J Public Health* 2005 Nov-Dec;96(6):406–408.

36. Fouchier R, Kuiken T, Rimmelzwaan G, Osterhaus A. Global task force for influenza. *Nature* 2005;435(7041):419–420.

37. Peiris JS, Lai ST, Poon LL, Guan Y, Yam LY, Lim W, Nicholls J, Yee WK, Yan WW, Cheung MT, Cheng VC, Chan KH, Tsang DN, Yung RW, Ng TK, Yuen KY, SARS Study Group. Coronavirus as a possible cause of severe acute respiratory syndrome. *Lancet* 2003;361(9366):1319–1325.

38. Drosten C, Gunther S, Preiser W, van der Werf S, Brodt HR, Becker S, Rabenau H, Panning M, Kolesnikova L, Fouchier RA, Berger A, Burguiere AM, Cinatl J, Eickmann M, Escriou N, Grywna K, Kramme S, Manuguerra JC, Muller S, Rickerts V, Sturmer M, Vieth S, Klenk HD, Osterhaus AD, Schmitz H, Doerr HW. Identification of a novel coronavirus in patients with severe acute respiratory syndrome. *N Engl J Med* 2003;348(20):1967–1976. Epub 2003 Apr 10.

39. Ksiazek TG, Erdman D, Goldsmith CS, Zaki SR, Peret T, Emery S, Tong S, Urbani C, Comer JA, Lim W, Rollin PE, Dowell SF, Ling AE, Humphrey CD, Shieh WJ, Guarner J, Paddock CD, Rota P, Fields B, DeRisi J, Yang JY, Cox N, Hughes JM, LeDuc JW, Bellini WJ, Anderson LJ, SARS Working Group. A novel coronavirus associated with severe acute respiratory syndrome. *N Engl J Med* 2003;348(20):1953–1966. Epub 2003 Apr 10.

40. Fouchier RA, Kuiken T, Schutten M, van Amerongen G, van Doornum GJ, van den Hoogen BG, Peiris M, Lim W, Stohr K, Osterhaus AD. Aetiology: Koch's postulates fulfilled for SARS virus. *Nature* 2003;423(6937):240.

41. Ferguson NM, Cummings DA, Cauchemez S, Fraser C, Riley S, Meeyai A, Iamsirithaworn S, Burke DS. Strategies for containing an emerging influenza pandemic in Southeast Asia. *Nature* 2005;437(7056):209–214. Epub 2005 Aug 3.

42. Longini IM Jr, Nizam A, Xu S, Ungchusak K, Hanshaoworakul W, Cummings DA, Halloran ME. Containing pandemic influenza at the source. *Science* 2005;309(5737):1083–1087. Epub 2005 Aug 3.

INTRODUCTION OF NEW AND UNDERUTILIZED VACCINES: PERSPECTIVES FROM THE AMERICAS

Jon Kim Andrus, MD,[1] *John Fitzsimmons, MURP,*[2]
and Ciro A. de Quadros, MD, MPH[3]

BACKGROUND

In this complex, ever-changing world, making new or old vaccines available to those children and families who most need them should be a top priority (1). The strategies of the Pan American Health Organization (PAHO) for introducing new and underutilized vaccines include three overriding, guiding principles: 1) increase access and equity, 2) accelerate disease control on a regional level, and 3) develop public health infrastructure. This chapter will present how these guiding principles have framed the lessons learned from introducing new vaccines in the Americas.

Equity emerges as a critical cross-cutting concept that drives much of the work of PAHO and member countries (2). In terms of vaccines, the persistent challenge is to ensure that every community benefits from the potential impact of these technologies. Reducing the availability gap of new vaccines in developing countries means fast-tracking the time usually required to get from research and development to actual introduction of the vaccines, which usually has taken between 10 and 15 years. The strategy to shorten this time frame should be coupled with efforts to negotiate affordable prices for all. This process also must embrace a perception that vaccines are one of the most effective public health interventions

---

[1] Lead Technical Advisor, Immunization Unit, Pan American Health Organization.
[2] Senior Program Officer, Immunization Unit, Pan American Health Organization.
[3] Director of International Programs, Albert A. Sabin Institute.

available. In many parts of the world, the value of vaccines is underappreciated, leading to insufficient support for vaccine development, production, and use (3).

In the Americas, efforts to control disease over the last 20 years have led to significant improvements in the public health infrastructure, particularly in program management, surveillance, and public health laboratories. In some countries, such as Brazil, the development of public sector capacity for vaccine production also has become a top priority (4). Such public sector capacity development leads to regional independence, competition among private sector producers that reduces vaccine prices, and dependable and sustainable supply chains that contribute to intercountry cooperation. Currently, Brazil produces yellow fever vaccine that has been used in (and in some cases donated to) neighboring countries experiencing yellow fever outbreaks.

To strengthen these efforts, sound policy decisions on new and underutilized vaccine introduction must address several factors including (5–8):

- disease burden data,
- characteristics of the new vaccine and its impact on program feasibility,
- overall perception of risk, including the public's perception of risk,
- economic analyses of interventions,
- vaccine supply,
- political commitment and support, and
- the creation of partnerships and their sustainability.

The information required to make sound policy decisions is part of a complete package that complements the scientific data generated from exhaustive pre-licensure research (9).

DISEASE BURDEN DATA

Recognizing that a vaccine-preventable disease is a public health problem, as demonstrated by the disease burden data, is an important first step in the process of policy development. When research and surveillance data are immediately available, the disease burden is easily recognized, thus facilitating policy development. Such was the case with measles elimination in the early 1990s (10). When a lack of sufficient data makes it difficult to estimate the disease burden, however—as was the case with congenital rubella syndrome (CRS)—policy making is undermined. This occurred prior to the launching of the measles elimination initiative in 1994, when only a few countries in the Region had introduced the rubella vaccine into their routine program (11).

In 1994, after polio was eradicated in the Americas, the recognition and understanding of measles morbidity and mortality led the ministries of health in the Region to adopt a measles elimination initiative by 2000 (*12*). In 1990, nearly 240,000 measles cases were reported in the Region of the Americas, but only 7,640 rubella cases and no cases of congenital rubella syndrome were reported. Prior to 1992, only four countries submitted reports for rubella cases; by 1998 all countries of the Region were reporting cases. By 1996, the reported measles cases in the Region had dipped to a record low of 2,109 (*13*). That same year, 95,010 cases of rubella were reported. By 1998, the Region reported 14,332 measles cases, 123,815 rubella cases, and 44 congenital rubella syndrome cases. Reporting of CRS cases began in 1998, and these cases are underreported. Improved understanding of rubella through surveillance of rash and fever for measles elimination led to an increase in the reported cases of rubella, exposing what had been a silent but deadly disease (*14*). Better congenital rubella syndrome surveillance in the Region is still needed to fully map the disease burden.

CHARACTERISTICS OF THE NEW VACCINE AND ITS IMPACT ON PROGRAM FEASIBILITY

Essential characteristics which need to be demonstrated before the introduction of new vaccines include:

- immunogenicity and efficacy,
- immunity duration,
- interaction with other antigens,
- safety and adverse event profile,
- dosage and route of administration, and
- storage and thermostability.

Immunogenicity may vary as a function of age or immune status. Polysaccharide vaccines are less immunogenic than their equivalent, more expensive, conjugate counterparts in infants and young children. In the Americas, efforts were successful in making the conjugate Hib vaccine affordable for use virtually in all countries (except in Haiti). The development of the septavalent conjugate vaccine to replace the less immunogenic pneumococcal polysaccharide vaccine used in the United States was a significant breakthrough, in that it provided better protection for children against pneumococcal disease. In the United States this vaccine was made available to all children, not just those living in high-risk areas. Although cholera is a major public health problem in many tropical areas of the world, vaccines against cholera have not been as efficacious. Consequently, strategies to control cholera do not rely on vaccination.

Vaccines that provide shorter periods of protection require frequent and more regular booster doses, as does the tetanus toxoid vaccine. Fortunately, tetanus toxoid vaccine is cheap and has had a profound impact on the morbidity and mortality associated with neonatal tetanus. Live vaccines have less of a problem with waning immunity, but often confer less than 100% protection. Recent experience in numerous countries has exposed the need for providing a second opportunity for measles vaccine to assure that protection is close to 100%. Rubella vaccine confers lifelong immunity and is operationally much easier to use for disease control. Other issues, such as herd immunity, may also influence the potential impact of a vaccine on disease control.

Dosage and route of administration are other important characteristics of a vaccine to be considered. Vaccines that can be easily integrated into a routine immunization schedule of children 2, 4, and 6 months of age (such as the rotavirus vaccine) are much more acceptable than those which require additional, non-routine visits to the health center (15). However, restrictions imposed by dosage requirements or thermogenicity issues may require exceptional storage capacity or lower temperature maintenance, making the incorporation of certain vaccines into national immunization programs operationally more difficult.

Clearly, a vaccine's characteristics are inextricably linked to issues that are relevant to the feasibility of programs. For example, the cold chain and the distribution system are critical components of program feasibility that must be addressed. Despite the fact that there may be widespread consensus for introducing a particular new vaccine, existing capacity may not be able to absorb the introduction unless logistical and infrastructure issues are considered. The elements of this capacity include, but are not limited to, availability of cold chain, trained staff, and post-marketing surveillance. When the pentavalent vaccine was introduced in the Americas, the Region's cold-chain capabilities were sufficient to rapidly absorb this new activity (16).

OVERALL RISK PERCEPTION, INCLUDING THE PUBLIC'S

Large industrialized countries tend to introduce new vaccines first, followed by middle and lower income countries. The perception of risk differs from country to country, and this may influence the process. Diphtheria-pertussis-tetanus combination toxoid vaccine (DPT) has long been one of the vaccines traditionally included in developing countries' Expanded Immunization Program (EPI). The impact of this life-saving vaccine against these three fatal childhood diseases has been remarkable. In fact, people may have forgotten how these killer diseases spread panic in communities during the pre-vaccine era outbreaks.

As the incidence of a given disease decreases with vaccination, the population begins to focus more on the vaccine's side effects and adverse events, and less on its benefits in terms of disease protection. When this happens in a country, many have argued that the greatest threat to success is resistance to continue vaccinating. The public needs to be reassured that vaccines are safe and that they represent good public health practice, and that, although rare, vaccine-related side-effects are rigorously followed and investigated (17).

In the United States, injury-compensation lawsuits and their costs led to the enactment of the Vaccine Injury Compensation Act (18). The act allowed families to be compensated for adverse events caused by vaccination, but put a ceiling on the amount. Prior to the act, compensation had escalated to such levels that the financial sustainability of the federal program was at risk. In 1997, the United States changed its policy from administering DTwP (containing whole-cell pertussis) to administering DTaP (acellular pertussis) (19, 20). This policy change was substantially influenced by the public's perception of risk of pertussis disease (acellular pertussis [PA] has fewer side effects than the traditional whole-cell vaccine used in DPT), as well as by the need to cut financial losses resulting from an increasingly litigious environment resulting in many lawsuits seeking injury compensation.

Latin American and Caribbean countries, on the other hand, still use the traditional whole-cell DPT. And, while the disease burden has been greatly reduced, sporadic outbreaks of diphtheria (Paraguay in 2003, Dominican Republic in 2004) (21, 22) and pertussis (El Salvador in 2005) still occur. The perception of risk in many of these lower income countries is influenced by the presence of natural infection and not by the rare serious side effects of the vaccines themselves. In addition, the litigious atmosphere that prevails in North American countries may not exist in Latin America and the Caribbean.

While perception of risk may be important, there also are sound scientific arguments for sustaining the use of whole-cell pertussis vaccines in countries that have periodic outbreaks. The efficacy achieved when using many DPT vaccines appears to be as good as or better than that attained with some DPaT vaccines (23). Cost is another influencing factor, and DPT is considerably cheaper. Given these aspects, as well as the need to maintain access and equity, PAHO recommends the use of pentavalent vaccine that contains diphtheria, whole-cell pertussis, tetanus, hepatitis B, and *Haemophilus influenzae* type b antigens.

VACCINE SUPPLY

Vaccines must be affordable if countries are to use them. But a vaccine's price also must be high enough to allow the manufacturer to recoup its development and manufacturing costs, and so guarantee supply, and low enough to allow a country with limited resources for health to be able to purchase it (24).

Prior to the creation of the PAHO Revolving Fund for Vaccine Procurement in the Americas, countries frequently ran out of critical vaccine inventories required to protect their children against killer diseases. The Revolving Fund established a mechanism whereby vaccine supply was stabilized and guaranteed for participating countries. The Fund allows PAHO to purchase vaccines on their behalf; the Organization does all the administrative work of negotiating affordable prices, drawing up contracts, placing orders, and ensuring the safe and timely delivery of orders. PAHO does this at a minimum charge of 3% to maintain capitalization of the Fund. Countries can purchase the vaccines assured that PAHO will take immediate action to make the vaccine available. They have 60 days to reimburse the Fund.

Accurate forecasting—measured by demand and available supply—is essential for manufacturers to plan for and produce required vaccines. The Revolving Fund works hard to maintain accurate demand forecasting, knowing that disruptions in demand adversely affect prices when produced vaccines are not off-loaded by producers. Intrinsically linked to demand is the public's acceptance of the vaccine, which may vary from country to country (25). This has certainly been the case in the incorporation of yellow fever vaccine in the Americas, where yearly outbreaks with associated high case-fatality rates continue to occur in tropical areas.

Some vaccines—influenza vaccine and pneumococcal conjugate vaccines are two—are more difficult to produce technologically, which decreases the capability of maintaining sufficient supplies of them. For example, each influenza vaccine dose requires one egg embryo to produce. Fortunately, newer technologies such as vero cell culture or genetic techniques may circumvent this impediment and allow for a sufficient supply to cover the entire world's population. The septavalent pneumococcal conjugate vaccine that is currently used in the United States comprises seven serotypes. The production of each serotype is as labor intensive as the production of a single vaccine, however.

ECONOMIC ANALYSES AND INTERVENTIONS

There are several tools available for assessing whether the investment in vaccines and immunization is worthwhile. The most useful among them are cost analysis, cost-benefit analysis, cost-effectiveness analysis, and cost-utility analyses. These sorts of analyses have consistently demonstrated that immunization is an excellent investment (26).

Cost-benefit analysis is useful for determining the overall balance of costs and benefits associated with a particular program. As do other types of analyses, cost-benefit analysis assigns a monetary value to all costs and all benefits of a policy or program. Benefits are calculated by estimating the total cost of the disease in the absence of intervention and subtracting from that the total costs of residual disease occurring with the program (27). This has been found useful when comparing health programs with non-health programs. In the Caribbean, for example, cost-benefit analysis determined that the elimination of congenital rubella syndrome would cost 7% of the total cost required to treat and rehabilitate cases of congenital rubella syndrome if they were to occur in the absence of an elimination program (27). These data were extremely useful in launching the rubella and congenital rubella syndrome elimination initiative in the Caribbean, the first such initiative in the Americas.

Cost-effectiveness analysis also is useful for determining how much an intervention costs to produce a particular outcome. The results of these analyses are expressed in terms of cost per case or death averted, or cost per life-year gained. Cost-effectiveness analysis also enables a comparison to be made of several strategies achieving a single effect. Cost-utility analysis is a specific form of cost-effectiveness analysis in which outcomes are distilled to a common denominator, such as disability-adjusted life year. In the case of the introduction of rotavirus vaccine in the Americas, we know that the cost per disability-adjusted life year gained is comparable to that achieved with breast-feeding (28). This has been tremendously useful in generating advocacy and interest for a vaccine that potentially could help address a very important public health problem in the Americas.

Ministers of health can grasp the scientific justification for introducing new vaccines as a way to close the equity gap and make these technologies available to those who most need them, but they must negotiate increased funding for them with their ministry of finance counterparts. Far too often, the risk of taking financial resources from one program sector to support another becomes an unfortunate reality. In this context, creating fiscal space will be a critical consideration. Creating fiscal space means identifying new revenue sources to finance the introduction of new and underutilized vaccines that do not compete with existing programs and without affecting macro-economic stability. The national lottery in Costa Rica and the National Health Fund in Jamaica (established through collection of "sin" taxes on tobacco and alcohol consumption) are excellent examples of new sources of revenue that can be shunted to finance immunization activities. Some countries also are considering how to improve the management of the existing tax administration systems to reduce tax evasion and collect more revenue to finance the expansion of social programs. In PAHO's case, Revolving Fund cost savings identified along its supply chain lead to gains in efficiency, creating more fiscal space within the sector (29).

POLITICAL COMMITMENT AND SUPPORT

There is much to be proud of with the progress made in childhood immunization programs worldwide, but this is not universally felt (30). The re-emergence of polio in 2004 and 2005 in Nigeria and elsewhere in the world is a good example of what can happen when the political commitment that sustains progress in the global polio eradication initiative lags (31).

Immunization is a right that must be protected through the political process. Political leaders recognize, more than ever, that childhood immunization is a cost-saving endeavor that returns much more to society than it costs. PAHO's Directing Council serves as the forum where all ministers of health in the Americas can discuss and develop Regionwide policies (32). Initiatives such as polio eradication and the elimination of measles and rubella were adopted. The recent introduction of rubella vaccine would have never occurred as a regional policy had it not been for the collective political commitment exhibited by the ministers of health. In 2003, again promoting access, accelerated disease control, and development of public health infrastructure, the Directing Council adopted the initiative to eliminate rubella and congenital rubella syndrome from the Americas by the year 2010. To maximize the impact of rubella elimination, countries are sharing experiences on how to use the initiative to improve women's health, the surveillance and follow-up of all congenital birth defects, and perinatal care in general (33).

Rotavirus disease is another example where political commitment has been critical for prioritizing public health interventions. Rotavirus outbreaks occur annually in Central American countries (34). In July 2004, PAHO, in partnership with the Albert B. Sabin Vaccine Institute and the United States Centers for Disease Control and Prevention, convened a technical meeting in Mexico City to review the epidemiologic situation and the development and introduction of a vaccine against rotavirus. Rotavirus kills nearly 16,000 children and causes more than 77,000 hospitalizations annually in the Americas. After reviewing these data, the country representatives attending this meeting decided to adopt a resolution to accelerate the introduction of rotavirus vaccine. This proclamation, called the Mexico City Resolution, has since served as an advocacy tool for enlisting support to address this important public health challenge (35). As was the case with the polio, measles, and rubella Regional initiatives, this commitment results from a groundswell of country-based activities and advocacy efforts.

FIGURE 1. Countries that have enacted vaccine legislation, Region of the Americas, 2005.

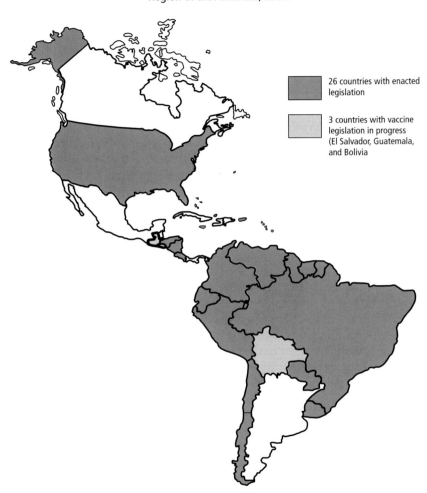

26 countries with enacted legislation

3 countries with vaccine legislation in progress (El Salvador, Guatemala, and Bolivia

Source: Country Reports to PAHO, as of April 2005.

Political commitment also has led to the development of legislative frameworks that help guarantee the sustainability of national immunization programs. In 2003, 19 countries had legislation stating that immunization services must be provided to the nation's children. This legislation served as a major step towards reducing inequities in immunization and health (36). By 2005, the number of countries with immunization-related legislation had increased to 26, and 3 others were in the process of enacting similar legislation (Figure 1). A comparative analysis of this legislation

TABLE 1. Analysis of vaccination legislation in selected countries in the Americas, 2005.

	Countries					
Key topics	Honduras	Ecuador	Paraguay	Venezuela	Costa Rica	Peru
Register facilitation						✔
Supply regulations					✔	
Custom clearance				✔		✔
Disbursement regulation		✔	✔		✔	
Contractual flexibility	✔	✔			✔	
Tax exemptions	✔			✔	✔	
Obligatory vaccination			✔	✔	✔	✔
Enforceability	✔		✔	✔	✔	
Vaccines at no cost[a]	✔		✔	✔	✔	✔
Budget line[b]	✔	✔	✔	✔	✔	✔
Year enacted	1998	1997	2003	1996	2001	2002

[a] Means that a country is committed to public good.
[b] Means that vaccination is a priority in the country.

Source: Immunization Unit, Pan American Health Organization.

across countries reveals that key topics relating to rationale, resources, acquisition, and vaccination may be identified at different levels within the process (Table 1). Vaccination as a public good and vaccination line items included in the national budget were the factors more commonly identified with good practice. Further analysis should help strengthen existing legislation and serve as a reference for countries considering new legislation in the future.

PARTNERSHIPS

A study evaluating the factors leading to policy decisions in countries found that the involvement of the community dealing with pediatric issues, particularly opinion leaders in that community, was essential to the process (37). The introduction of pentavalent vaccine in the countries of the Americas was also driven by a similar process. Key pediatricians and pediatric societies supported improved surveillance of bacterial invasive disease, which led to a better understanding of Hib disease prevalence in the countries (16). Other related surveillance and disease-burden issues included the need to better understand the development of antimicrobial resistance. Chile, the United States, and Uruguay had introduced Hib vaccine and were able to demonstrate a significant reduction in disease incidence. These experiences served as a springboard for promoting the introduction of *Haemophilus influenzae* type b vaccine by ministries of health of other countries, supported by the pediatric provider community.

SUMMARY

PAHO's strategy in support of the introduction of new and underutilized vaccines into national immunization programs in the Americas is multi-faceted. It is directed toward strengthening available information so that policy makers and public health professionals can make sound decisions. The introduction of new and underutilized vaccines is guided by principles of equity in access to the services that deliver the vaccine, as well as an effort to accelerate the control of the target disease while assuring that the mode of introduction of the vaccine strengthens public health infrastructure. This has been the pattern for the introduction of Hib-containing vaccines, principally pentavalent DTP-HepB-Hib, and will remain the model for the introduction of other new and underutilized vaccines. Reaching targets for child mortality reduction also requires that the introduction of new vaccines be consistent with overall national health policy and budget priorities. To this end, PAHO's support to countries emphasizes the development and use of evidence to guide new vaccine introduction decisions, including the use of disease-burden data and the conduct of cost-effectiveness and economic analyses.

References

1. Andrus JK, Fitzsimmons J. Introduction of new and underutilized vaccines: Sustaining access, disease control and infrastructure development. PLoS 2005. 2005;2(10):E286, 0101-2.
2. Andrus JK, Roses Periago M. Elimination of rubella and congenital rubella syndrome in the Americas: another opportunity to address inequities in health. *Rev Panam Salud Publica* (editorial) 2004;15(3):145–146.
3. Hausdorff WP. Prospects for the use of new vaccines in developing countries: cost is not the only impediment. *Vaccine* 1996;14(3):1179–1186.
4. Mahoney RT, Maynard JE. The introduction of new vaccines into developing countries. *Vaccine* 1999;17:646–652.
5. Andrus JK, Tambini G, di Fabio JL, Roses Periago M. Anticipating new vaccines in the Americas. *Rev Panam Salud Publica* 2004;16(6):369–370.
6. World Health Organization. Introduction of hepatitis B vaccine into childhood immunization services: management guidelines, including information for health workers and parents. Geneva: WHO, 2001.
7. World Health Organization. Introduction of *Haemophilus influenzae* type b vaccine into immunization programmes: management guidelines, including information for health workers and parents. Geneva: WHO, 2000.

8. Aylward B, Kane M, Batson A, McNair R. A framework for the evaluation of vaccines for use in the Expanded Programme of Immunization. *Vaccine* 1994; 12:1155–1159.
9. Clemens JD. Thinking downstream to accelerate the introduction of new vaccines for developing countries. *Vaccine* 2003;21:S2/114–S2/115.
10. Andrus JK, de Quadros CA. Global access: deployment, use, and acceptance. In: Khan P, Gust I, Koff W, eds. *Accelerating AIDS vaccine development: challenges and opportunities*. Norfolk, United Kingdom: Horizon Scientific Press (In press).
11. De Quadros CA, Izurieta H, Venczel L, Carrasco P. Measles eradication in the Americas: progress to date. *J Infect Dis* 2004;189(suppl 1):S227–S235.
12. Castillo-Solorzano C, Carrasco P, Tambini G, Reef S, Brana M, de Quadros CA. New horizons in control of rubella and congenital rubella syndrome in the Americas. *J Infect Dis* 2003;187:S146–S152.
13. Pan American Health Organization. Final Measles Surveillance Data, 1996. Special Program for Vaccines and Immunization Expanded Program on Immunization.
14. Pan American Health Organization. Measles elimination by the year 2000. *EPI Newsletter* 1994;16:1–2.
15. Halsey N. Practical considerations regarding the impact on immunization schedules of introduction of new combined vaccines. *Ann NY Acad Sci* 1995; 754:250.
16. Ropero AM, Danovaro-Holiday MC. Andrus JK. Progress in vaccination against hepatitis B in the Americas. *J Clin Virol* 2005 (In print).
17. Salisbury DM, Beverley PCL, Miller E. Vaccine programs and policy. *Br Med Bull* 2002;262:201–211.
18. Brink EW, Hinman AR. The Vaccine Injury Compensation Act: the new law and you. *Contemp Pediatr* July 1989;6(3):28–32, 35–36, 39, 42.
19. Centers for Disease Control and Prevention. Pertussis vaccination: use of acellular pertussis vaccines among infants and young children—recommendations of the Advisory Committee on Immunization Practices (ACIP). *MMWR* 1997;46(No. RR-7):2, 25.
20. Centers for Disease Control and Prevention. Notice to readers: recommended childhood immunization schedule—United States, 1997. *MMWR* 1997;46(02): 35–39.
21. Pan American Health Organization. Diphtheria outbreak in Paraguay. *EPI Newsletter* 2002;24(3):6.
22. Pan American Health Organization. Diphtheria outbreak in the Dominican Republic. *EPI Newsletter* 2002;26(3):1.
23. Edwards KM, Decker MD. Pertussis vaccine. In: Plotkin SA, Orenstein WA, eds. *Vaccines*, 4th ed. Philadelphia: WB Saunders Co, 2004:509.
24. Offit P. Why are pharmaceutical companies gradually abandoning vaccines? *Health Aff* 2005;24(3):622–630.
25. Streefland PH. Introduction of a HIV vaccine in developing countries: social and cultural dimensions. *Vaccine* 2002;21:1304–1309.
26. Hinman AR. Economic aspects of vaccines and immunization. *Life Sciences* 1999;322:989–994.

27. Hinman AR, Irons B, Lewis M, Kandola K. Economic analyses of rubella and rubella vaccines: a global review. *Bull WHO* 2002;80(4):264–270.
28. Podewils LJ, Antil L, Hummelman E, Bresee J, Parashar UD, Rheingans R. Projected cost-effectiveness of rotavirus vaccination for children in Asia. *J Infect Dis* 2005;192(suppl 1):X133–X145.
29. Stotsky JG, WoldeMariam A. Central American Tax Reform: Trends and Possibilities, IMF Working Papers 02/227. International Monetary Fund, 2002: 35–37.
30. Hinman AR. Immunization, equity, and human rights. *Am J Prev Med* 2004; 26(1):84–88.
31. Aylward, RB, Heymann DL. Can we capitalize on the virtues of vaccines? Insights from the polio eradication initiative. *Am J Public Health* 2005;95(5): 773–777.
32. Tambini G, Andrus JK, Fitzsimmons JW, Roses Periago M. Regional programs for health: immunization as a model for strengthening inter-country cooperation and control of infectious diseases. *Rev Panam Salud Publica* 2006;20(1): 54–59.
33. Castillo-Solorzano C, Andrus JK. Rubella elimination and improving health care for women. *Emerg Infect Dis* 2004;10(11):2017–2021.
34. Pan American Health Organization. Rotavirus update. *EPI Newsletter* 2005; 27(3):1.
35. Pan American Health Organization. Regional meeting for the Americas assesses progress against rotavirus. *Rev Panam Salud Publica* 2004;15(1):66–69.
36. Pan American Health Organization. Paraguay passes vaccine law. *EPI Newsletter* 2003;25(6):6–8.
37. Wenger JD, di Fabio J-L, Landaverde JM, Levine OS, Gaafar T. Introduction of Hib conjugate vaccines in the non-industrialized world: experience in four 'newly adopting' countries. *Vaccine* 1999;18:736–742.

RECENT DEVELOPMENTS WITH PROPHYLACTIC HUMAN PAPILLOMAVIRUS VACCINES

Merle Lewis, DrPH, MPH,[1] *and Felicity Cutts, MD, MSc, MBChB*[2]

HUMAN PAPILLOMAVIRUSES

One of the most important findings in cancer biology in the last quarter of the 20th century is evidence that infection of the lower genital tract with specific "high-risk" types of human papillomaviruses (HPV) causes virtually all cases of cervical carcinoma in women. Evidence also links these infections etiologically with a smaller, less defined fraction of vulvar, vaginal, anal, and penile cancers. For two decades, many epidemiological, clinical, and molecular-biology studies have confirmed HPV as the necessary and possibly sufficient cause of cervical neoplasia (1–7). These significant advances, along with a better understanding of the immunobiology of these viruses, paved the way for the subsequent development of vaccines, thus providing an exceptional opportunity for cervical cancer prevention through vaccination (8, 9).

Human papillomaviruses are small, non-enveloped, double-stranded DNA viruses that infect humans exclusively. They are entirely epitheliotropic, infecting the skin or the anogenital and oropharyngeal mucosa (10–12). The most frequently associated HPV lesions are warts, which can be flat (subclinical), papular, or cauliflower-like. Roughly 70% of HPV infections resolve spontaneously without clinical manifestations, and it has

[1] Regional Advisor on Vaccine Research and Development, Immunization Unit, Pan American Health Organization.
[2] Scientist, Initiative on Vaccine Research; Immunizations, Vaccines and Biologicals; World Health Organization.

been estimated that the median duration of these transient infections can range from about five to eight months, depending on the infecting virus type. Sometimes cervical HPV infections can persist, however, inducing cytologic abnormalities which can progressively worsen and lead to malignant changes. Persistent infection, usually defined as the presence of the same HPV DNA in cervicovaginal specimens on two or more occasions at least six months apart in women who were negative for the relevant type at baseline, is considered to indicate a high risk of progression to high-grade dysplasia and cervical cancer (13, 14).

Nearly 100 HPVs have been completely sequenced and characterized; 40 of them are known to primarily infect the genital epithelium (15). On the basis of extensive molecular epidemiological evidence, these genital HPVs have been subdivided into low-risk and high-risk oncogenic types. Low-risk types such as HPV 6 and HPV 11 cause about 90% of cases of genital warts (*Condylomata acuminata*), which occur on external surfaces of the vulva, anus, and vagina. The high-risk, oncogenic types, of which there are at least 13 (16, 18, 31, 33, 35, 39, 45, 51, 52, 56, 58, 59, 68), are associated with invasive cervical cancer (7). Of these, HPV 16 is by far the most common, being present in roughly half of cervical cancers worldwide; type 18 is the next most common, causing about 17% of the global cervical cancer burden. In Latin America and the Caribbean, virus types 45, 33, and 31 are also important causes of cervical cancer (7, 15–17). Although HPV type 18 accounts for fewer squamous cell cervical cancers than HPV 16, it causes a higher proportion of adenocarcinomas, even though the precise mechanism of HPV type-specific cellular tropism is unknown (12).

THE CERVICAL CANCER BURDEN

From a public health perspective, cervical cancer is the most important sequela of an HPV infection. This disease is a devastating health problem— it is the second most commonly occurring cancer among women worldwide and the leading female malignancy in the developing world. The World Health Organization and the International Agency for Research in Cancer (IARC) estimate that each year nearly half a million new cases and more than 230,000 deaths occur worldwide, with women in less developed countries bearing approximately 80% of the global cervical cancer burden (18, 19).

It has been estimated that 92,136 new cases and 37,640 deaths occur in the Americas each year due to this malignant neoplasm. Latin America and the Caribbean contribute 84% and 81% of the total estimated cases and deaths, respectively (18). When disease burden is measured in "disability-adjusted life-years" (DALYs), recent WHO estimates suggest that cervical cancer now accounts for 3.28 million DALYs globally and 502,000 DALYs in the Americas (19).

It is important to emphasize that, in addition to cases of invasive cervical cancer, estimates of the total HPV burden of severe disease should also include other HPV-related cancers (vulvar, penile, anal, oral cavity and tonsils) and the rare recurrent respiratory papillomatosis. In economic and social terms, much of the HPV-associated burden is borne by women with high- and low-grade cervical intraepithelial lesions, as well as those with HPV infections without evidence of cytological abnormalities. These women usually require extensive follow-up cytology, virology, colposcopy, and histology medical services, depending on the indication. The IARC has estimated that every year there are 300 million new HPV infections in women without evidence of cytologic cervical abnormalities, 30 million low-grade dysplasias (cervical intraepithelial neoplasia grade 1 [CIN1], and 10 million high-grade dysplasias [CIN2 and CIN3]) (20). In the United States, where approximately 50 million Papanicolaou smear tests are performed annually, 1.2 million cases of low-grade dysplasia, 300,000 cases of high-grade dysplasia, and 10,000 cases of cervical cancer are identified each year (21).

SECONDARY CERVICAL CANCER PREVENTION

For the last 50 years, effective secondary prevention of cervical cancer has been possible through screening with the Papanicolaou smear. In the United States, cervical cancer rates have plummeted by 75% since the Pap smear was introduced more than 40 years ago (22). In several European countries, the redirection of screening into organized, population-based programs with systems for call and recall of women has resulted in reductions between 25% and 30% higher than rates achieved through opportunistic screening (23). More recently, reports from Valdivia, Chile, note that a sustained increase of nearly 80% in screening coverage between 1993 and 2003 has reduced cervical cancer morbidity and mortality to such an extent that deaths in women 15 years old and older have dropped sharply from 18.9 per 100,000 in 1993 to 4.6 per 100,000 in 2003 (24).

In low-income, developing countries—including many Latin American and Caribbean countries—cervical cancer prevention programs have not generally resulted in the profound reductions in morbidity and mortality observed in industrialized countries of Europe and North America (25). The reasons for this are multi-faceted, relating in part to (a) the under-recognition of cervical cancer as a preventable public health problem; (b) the suboptimal management and coordination of prevention and control programs; (c) the fact that the necessary infrastructure resources to guarantee quality service along every point of the cancer care continuum have not been adequately sustained; and (d) the special sociocultural challenges women face (26). There are also inherent limitations in the Pap test: a single conventional cervical smear misses between 40% and 50% of biopsy-confirmed, high-grade cancer precursors and cervical cancers (25). This relative insensitivity demands that frequent testing be performed for optimal cancer protection, in turn compromising cost-efficiency and reducing the potential for client compliance with timely screening.

Traditional cervical cancer prevention and control programs based on screening, diagnosis, and treatment have also been very costly. In 2001, Costa Rica reported investments in cervical cancer programs that exceeded US$ 86 million (26); in the United States, the total health care cost associated with screening and treatment of cervical cancer is estimated to be US$ 6 billion per year (21, 27).

Given this background of high program costs, quality issues, and sociocultural challenges for secondary prevention, an HPV vaccine would be a welcomed primary preventive tool that could significantly enhance the prospects for comprehensive cervical cancer control.

HPV VACCINE DEVELOPMENT

To date, HPV vaccine development has progressed along two lines: as prophylactic vaccines to prevent first occurrences of HPV infections and as therapeutic vaccines to induce viral clearance and regression of existing pre-cancerous lesions. The development of a therapeutic HPV vaccine would be highly desirable for the estimated five million women worldwide already infected with HPV, but progress with therapeutic vaccines has lagged behind advances in prophylactic vaccines. This chapter will focus on the latter.

PROPHYLACTIC HPV VACCINES

Live attenuated or inactivated virions have been successfully used to develop effective prophylactic vaccines against infections such as poliomyelitis, measles, and yellow fever. These strategies were not available for HPV vaccine development for two important reasons. First, because HPVs are DNA tumor viruses that contain oncogenes, there is the theoretical argument that the presence of such genes in a vaccine could disrupt normal cell growth controls and result in vaccine-induced carcinogenesis. Second, because virus replication and assembly are tightly linked to the differentiation program of epithelial cells (infectious virions are produced only in the terminally differentiated cells and are shed as virus-laden squamous cells), it has not been possible to propagate HPV through the usually employed monolayer cell culture methods, thus precluding large-scale production. As a result, HPV vaccine development has been pursued through a subunit approach in which the vaccine is composed solely of a major capsid protein, L1, which has the intrinsic capacity to self-assemble into virus-like particles (VLPs) that are morphologically indistinguishable from authentic virions. The HPV L1 polypeptide of the relevant genotypes is expressed in recombinant yeast (*Saccharomyces cerevisiae*) or baculovirus vectors. In animal studies (*28*) as well as in Phase 1 studies in human volunteers, L1 VLPs were shown to induce the production of high titers of type-specific neutralizing IgG antibodies, which prevented infection with the relevant type upon subsequent exposure (*29*).

In 2001, it was reported that three doses of an HPV-16 L1-VLP vaccine, administered intramuscularly to 72 healthy HIV-seronegative volunteers aged 18–29 years, were well tolerated and highly immunogenic even without adjuvant. The majority of vaccine recipients achieved serum antibody titers that were approximately 40-fold higher than those observed in naturally acquired infections. In this double-blind, randomized, placebo-controlled, Phase 1 trial to evaluate the safety and immunogenicity of an HPV vaccine, the most commonly reported side effect was pain at the injection site. The pain was mild and short-lived, consistent with other intramuscularly administered recombinant subunit vaccines, such as licensed hepatitis B vaccine.

In a landmark study published in 2002, Koutsky and her colleagues reported on the findings of a double-blind, randomized, multi-center Phase II clinical trial, which was conducted in the United States using an HPV 16 L1-VLP vaccine. The study population consisted of 2,392 women aged 16–23 years, who were both HPV 16 DNA negative and antibody negative at enrollment. Women were randomly assigned to receive 0.5 ml of either placebo or vaccine administered intramuscularly at day 0, month 2, and month 6. Each vaccine dose contained 40 μg of HPV 16 L1 virus-like particles formulated on an aluminum adjuvant. The vaccine was shown to be 100% effective (95% CI: 90–100) in preventing persistent HPV infection, with no cases occurring among vaccinated women and 41 cases occurring in the placebo group, 9 of which were associated with cervical dysplasia of low or high grade (*30*).

Following on the success of the proof-of-principle study with monovalent HPV-16 vaccine, the Merck Company has developed and evaluated a quadrivalent HPV vaccine (6, 11, 16, and 18) in multicenter studies in North America, Brazil, and Europe. Results of the Phase II study, which were reported in 2005, showed 88% (95% CI: 72–96) protection against persistent infection associated with the four HPV types contained in the vaccine among women vaccinated in the intention-to-treat cohort (*31*) (Table 1). Results of the Phase III trials of the Merck vaccine were announced at the end of 2005, and they demonstrated 100% protection against CIN-2 or worse, with no cases occurring among vaccinees, as compared to 21 cases among placebo recipients among women fully vaccinated according to protocol (*32*). A recently presented combined analysis of three trials of the Merck product established vaccine efficacy against CIN-2, CIN-3, and adenocarcinoma in situ at 100% (*33*) (Table 2).

The GlaxoSmithKline (GSK) vaccine, containing types 16 and 18, is being evaluated in multicenter trials and in a population-based trial in Costa Rica. In 2004, Harper and her associates reported the findings of a Phase II trial conducted among 1,113 women aged 15–25 years in Brazil, Canada, and the United States, utilizing an HPV 16–18 L1 VLP vaccine (*34*). This vaccine was delivered with an adjuvant, ASO4, in a three-dose schedule at months 0, 1, and 6. This bivalent vaccine was demonstrated to be generally safe, well-tolerated, and highly immunogenic, with a vaccine efficacy of 100% (95% CI: 76.8–100) against persistent infection with HPV 16 and 18 genotypes in the according-to-protocol population. Vaccine efficacy against cervical cytological abnormalities of any stage, including atypical squamous cells of uncertain significance associated with HPV 16–18 infections, was recorded at 92.9% (95% CI: 70–98.3) based on the intention-to-treat analyses. The vaccine also induced antibody levels 80–100-fold higher than those elicited by natural infection. Results of extended follow-up of the women in this study show that protection is sustained up to a mean of 47 months post-vaccination (Table 2). Efficacy against persistent infection occurring at any time after the third dose of vaccine was 96% (95% CI: 75.2–99.9). While not statistically powered to measure efficacy against CIN 2+, this follow-up study reported an efficacy of 100% (95% CI: –7.7–100) against moderate or severe cervical dysplasia, with no cases occurring among vaccine recipients and only five cases occurring in the placebo group. Interestingly, the authors also found evidence of cross-protection against incident infection with type 31 or 45, which are closely related to types 16 and 18, respectively. Protection against persistent infection with these types has not yet been reported (*35*).

To summarize, the results of the trials undertaken to date demonstrate that these prophylactic vaccines are highly efficacious against persistent HPV infection; are able to reduce the incidence of type-specific associated cervical abnormalities; are well tolerated by subjects; and elicit very high, sustained humoral antibody responses at levels higher than those observed in natural infections. Systemic immunization with a sub-unit VLP HPV vaccine, even without adjuvant, can induce protective immunity against a sexually transmitted mucosal viral infection.

TABLE 1. Characteristics of two prophylactic candidate HPV vaccines and results of their vaccine trials.

Characteristics	Vaccines and trial results	
	Quadrivalent Merck vaccine	Bivalent GlaxoSmithKline vaccine
Virus-like particles (VLPs) of genotypes	6, 11, 16, 18	16, 18
Substrate	Yeast (*S. cerevisiae*)	Baculovirus-infected insect cells
Adjuvant	Alum (amorphous aluminum hydroxyphosphate sulphate)	ASO4 (aluminum hydroxide and monophosphoryl lipid A)
Dosing regimen	0, 2, 6 months	0, 1, 6 months
Countries/regions included in reported vaccine evaluation	Brazil (34%); Europe (21%); USA (45%)	Brazil and North America (over 50% of women were from Brazil)
Antibody responses to type 16 in vaccinees compared to natural infection	260-fold higher at peak; 35-fold higher at 36 months post-vaccination	Over 100-fold higher at peak; 17-fold higher at 51–53 months post-vaccination
Antibody responses to type 18 in vaccinees compared to natural infection	67-fold higher at peak; 6-fold higher at 36 months	Over 80-fold higher at peak; 14-fold higher at 51–53 months post-vaccination
Number of cases in vaccine and placebo groups and VE (vaccine efficacy) (95% CI) against persistent infection (assessed in samples 4–6 apart) due to vaccine types	6 versus 47 cases VE-88 % (72–96) up to 36 months	2 versus 34 cases VE-94.4 % (78.2–99.4)
Number of cases in vaccine and placebo groups and VE against CIN (cervical intraepithelial neoplasia) (Merck) or ASCUS (atypical squamous cells of undetermined significance)/CIN (GSK) due to vaccine types	0 versus 7 cases VE-100% (32–100)	2 versus 44 VE-95.7% (83.5–99.5)
Cross-protection	Not yet reported	Significant reduction in incident infection with type 45 VE-94.2% (63.3–99.9) and type 31 VE-54.5% (11.5–77.7)

Sources: Villa LL, Costa RLR, Petta CA, Andrade RP et al. Prophylactic quadrivalent human papillomavirus [types 6, 11, 16 and 18] L1virus-like particle vaccine in young women: a randomized double-blind placebo-controlled multicentre phase 11 efficacy trial. *Lancet* 6:271–278, 2005. Harper DM, EL Franco, C Wheeler, DG Ferris, et al. Efficacy of a bivalent L1-virus-like particle vaccine in prevention of infection with human papillomavirus types 16 and 18 in young women: a randomized controlled trial. *Lancet* 364:1757–1765, 2004. Harper DM, EL Franco, CM Wheeler, AB Mosciki, et al. Sustained efficacy up to 4.5 years of a bivalent L1 virus-like particle vaccine against human papillomavirus types 16 and 18: follow-up from a randomized control trial. *Lancet* 367:1247–1255, 2006. (Available at http://www.thelancet.com April 15, 2006.)

TABLE 2. Updated characteristics of the licensed quadrivalent Merck vaccine.

Characteristics	Quadrivalent Merck vaccine	Data sources
Number of cases in vaccine and placebo groups and VE (vaccine efficacy) (95% CI) against persistent infection due to vaccine types	2 versus 46 cases VE-96% (84–100) up to 60 months	Abstract presented by Villa et al.[1] at the Meeting of the European Research Organization on Genital Infection and Neoplasia [EUROGIN], April 2006, Paris, France
Number of cases in vaccine and placebo groups and VE against cervical or genital lesions due to vaccine types	1 versus 113 cases VE-99% (95–100) against genital warts and vulvar and vaginal intraepithelial neoplasia of any grade	Abstract presented by Luisa Villa[2] on behalf of the Future II Study Group at the Meeting of the European Research Organization on Genital Infection and Neoplasia (EUROGIN), April 2006, Paris, France
Number of cases in vaccine and placebo groups and VE against cervical intraepithelial neoplasia (CIN) 2 + OR AIS (adenocarcinoma in situ)	0 versus 36 cases VE versus CIN2 – 100% (89–100) 0 versus 53 cases VE versus CIN2-3+ – 100% (93–100) 0 versus 32 cases VE versus CIN3 or AIS – 100% (88–100)	Abstract presented by Kevin Ault[3] at the European Cancer Conference (ECCO 13), 30 October–3 November 2005, Paris, France
Number of cases in vaccine and placebo groups and VE against vulvar intraepithelial neoplasia (VIN) 2/3 or vaginal intraepithelial neoplasia (VaIN) 2/3	0 versus 10 cases VE against VIN 2–3 or VaIN 2–3 – 100% (56–100)	Abstract presented by J. Paavonen[4] at the 2006 Annual Meeting of the American Society of Clinical Oncologists (ASCO), June 2006, USA

[1] Efficacy of a prophylactic quadrivalent human papillomavirus (HPV) types 6/11/16/18 L1 virus-like particle (VLP) vaccine through up to 5 years of follow-up.
[2] Efficacy of a quadrivalent HPV (types 6, 11, 16, 18) L1 VLP vaccine against external genital disease: a combined analysis.
[3] Prophylactic use of quadrivalent human papillomavirus (HPV) (types 6, 11, 16, 18) L1 virus-like particle (VLP) vaccine reduces cervical intraepithelial neoplasia (CIN) 2/3 and adenocarcinoma in situ (AIS) risk.
[4] Efficacy of a quadrivalent HPV (types 6/11/16/18) L1 virus-like particle (VLP) vaccine against vaginal and vulvar precancerous lesions: a combined analysis.

The publication of results from the international Phase III trials is expected soon. As discussed earlier, the quadrivalent HPV 16, 18, 11, 6 vaccine has been tested in 25,000 subjects in an international Phase III trial, in which Peru, Mexico, Brazil, and Colombia are participating from Latin America. The bivalent HPV 16–18 VLP vaccine is being tested in 90 centers in 14 countries (including Brazil and Mexico) among 13,000 women aged 15–25 years, as well as in a population-based trial in Guanacaste, Costa Rica. Prevention of high-grade precancerous dysplasia associated with a vaccine type is the primary endpoint in these Phase III trials; prevention of persistent HPV infection will also be evaluated. In June 2006, the quadrivalent HPV vaccine was licensed both in Mexico and the United States for use in women aged 9–26 years.

HPV VACCINE COST-EFFECTIVENESS

Rational planning for comprehensive cervical cancer prevention requires, among other important inputs, information on the cost-effectiveness of both the primary and secondary preventive interventions and of others that might be available. Much information on the cost-effectiveness of cervical cancer screening already exists in the published literature. For example, based on data from five low- and middle-income countries, including Peru, Goldie and colleagues have estimated that screening and treatment can be highly cost-effective when using appropriate techniques designed to optimize efficiency (36). Screening women once at age 35 years, utilizing visual inspection of the cervix with acetic acid, or performing DNA testing for human papillomavirus in cervical cell samples reduced the lifetime risk of cancer by approximately 25% to 36% and cost less than US$ 500 per year of life saved. Reductions of more than twice that could be achieved by two screenings at ages 35 and 40 years, while still remaining within the estimated cost per year of life saved that is considered to be highly cost-effective. These models (36–38) are now being extended to incorporate estimation of the effect of HPV vaccination (39–41). In general, all of these studies have established that a program of HPV vaccination that allows for a later initiation of screening and less frequent screening intervals is likely to be a cost-effective use of health care resources in countries with established screening programs (38).

In the United States, a mathematical simulation model demonstrated that HPV vaccination of 12-year-old girls would improve life expectancy at a marginal cost of US$ 246 relative to current practice, for an incremental cost-effectiveness ratio of $22,755 per extra quality-adjusted life year (QALY) gained. This model postulates that vaccination of the current cohort of 12-year-old girls (approximately 1,988,600) in the United States would avert more than 224,255 cases of HPV, 112,710 cases of squamous intraepithelial lesions, 3,317 cases of cervical cancer, and 1,340 cervical cancer deaths over the lifetime of this cohort (39). Another model has estimated that the most effective strategy with an incremental cost-effectiveness ratio of less than US$ 60,000 per QALY is one combining vaccination at age 12 years with triennial conventional cytologic screening beginning at age 25.

Such a strategy would reduce the absolute lifetime risk of cervical cancer by 94%, as compared with no intervention (40). In a third model, vaccination combined with biennial screening delayed until age 24 years yielded the most attractive cost-effectiveness ratio of US $44,889 per life year saved compared with screening only beginning at age 18 and conducted every three years (41).

Work is ongoing to estimate the cost-effectiveness of various strategies: vaccination alone, screening alone, or vaccination plus screening in resource constrained settings. It is anticipated that these cost-effectiveness models will be further refined as more results become available on the transmission dynamics of HPV infection, the program costs and effectiveness of different screening and treatment modalities and algorithms in developing countries, the cost of the vaccine, the duration of protection, and whether or not there is a need for boosters (42).

CONCLUSIONS

Prophylactic HPV vaccines have shown unprecedented levels of protection against new and persistent HPV infection and, in preliminary results to date, against related high-grade cervical lesions. Thus, these vaccines hold great promise for preventing cervical cancer. Despite the tremendous progress achieved to date in the development of HPV vaccines to prevent cervical cancer, several outstanding issues remain (40). One of these relates to the unknown duration of immunity induced by these L1-VLP vaccines. Preliminary data from several Phase II trials have indicated that antibody titers fall by about one log from peak levels achieved after immunization, reach a plateau about 18 months after vaccination, and persist at levels several-fold higher than those following natural infection for at least 47 months post-vaccination. Other questions include vaccine safety and efficacy in HIV-infected persons, coadministration with other vaccines, safety and immunogenicity in populations such as those in Africa that have not been included in trials to date, the degree of flexibility in the primary schedule in terms of intervals between each dose, the potential to vaccinate earlier than 9 years of age (the youngest age included in trials to date), and the degree of cross-protection against persistent infection and associated lesions with other high-risk types. The predicted cost-effectiveness of HPV vaccination, combined with secondary prevention, needs to be determined in different settings.

There are also many programmatic and sociocultural challenges associated with the future introduction of a vaccine whose primary target age group is likely to be young adolescents (43). Intersectoral linkages and partnerships will be needed to provide education and advocacy for HPV vaccination. Some countries may elect to vaccinate older adolescents and young women in addition to the primary target group.

Although there is great optimism for the introduction of HPV vaccines for the primary prevention of cervical cancer, it will be critical to continue to emphasize that secondary prevention through screening must still be available for women, since the vaccine will not protect against all high-risk cervical cancer-causing types. It is also unlikely that the vaccine will prevent cancer in women who have already been infected with the high-risk types included in the vaccine. Because cervical cancer screening is a cost-effective secondary prevention method, countries with functional screening programs will need to define the role of these in monitoring and evaluating HPV vaccination.

References

1. Zur Hausen H. Papillomaviruses in human cancers. *Proc Assoc Am Physicians* 1999;111:581–587.
2. Walboomers JMM, Jacobs MV, Manos MM, et al. Human papillomavirus is a necessary cause of invasive cervical cancer worldwide. *J Pathol* 1999;189: 12–19.
3. Munoz N. Human papillomavirus and cancer: the epidemiologic evidence. *J Clin Virol* 2000;19(1–2):1–5.
4. Bosch FX, Lorincz A, Munoz N, Meijer CJ, Shah KV. The causal relation between human papillomavirus and cervical cancer. *J Clin Pathol* 2002;55: 244–265.
5. Bosch FX, de Sanjose S. Human papillomavirus and cervical cancer—burden and assessment of causality. *J Natl Cancer Inst Monogr* 2003;31:3–13.
6. Schiffman M, Kjaer SK. Natural history of anogenital papillomavirus infection and neoplasia. *J Natl Cancer Inst Monogr* 2003;31:14–19.
7. Munoz, N, Bosch FX, de Sanjose S, Herrero R, et al. Epidemiologic classification of human papillomavirus types associated with cervical cancer. *N Engl J Med* 2003;348(6):518–527.
8. Schiller JT, Lowy DR. Human papillomavirus vaccines for cervical cancer prevention. In: Plotkin SA, Orenstein, WA, eds. *Vaccines*. Amsterdam: Elsevier Saunders, 2004:1259–1265.
9. Stanley MA. Human papillomavirus (HPV) vaccines: prospects for eradicating cervical cancer. *J Fam Plann Reprod Health Care* 2004;30(4):213–215.
10. Howley PM. Papillomavirinae: the viruses and their replication. In: Fields BN, Knipe DM, Howley PM, eds. *Fields virology*. Philadelphia: Lippincott-Raven, 1996:2045–2076.
11. Shah KV, Howley PM. Papillomaviruses. In: Fields BN, DM Knipe, PM Howley (eds.) *Fields Virology*. Philadelphia (PA): Lippincott-Raven; 1996: 2077–2109.
12. Stoler MH. Human papillomavirus biology and cervical neoplasia: implications for diagnostic criteria and testing. *Arch Pathol Lab Med* 2003;127(8): 935–939.

13. Ho GY, Bierman R, Beardsley L, et al. Natural history of cervico-vaginal papillomavirus infection in young women. *N Engl J Med* 1998;338:1365–1371.
14. Schlecht NF, Platt RW, Negassa A, Duarte-Franco E, et al. Modelling the time dependence of the association between human papillomavirus infection and cervical cancer precursor lesions. *Am J Epidemiol* 2003;158:878–886.
15. Schiffman MH, Burk RD. Human papillomaviruses. In: Evans AS, Kaslow RA, eds. *Viral infections in humans—epidemiology and control*, 4th ed. New York: Plenum Medical Book Company; 1997.
16. Bosch FX, Manos MM, Munoz N, Sherman M, et al. Prevalence of human papillomavirus in cervical cancer: a worldwide perspective. International Biological Study on Cervical Cancer [IBSCC] Study Group. *J Natl Cancer Inst* 1995;87(11):796–802.
17. Clifford GM, Smith JS, Plummer M, Munoz N, et al. Human papillomavirus types in invasive cervical cancer worldwide: a meta-analysis. *Br J Cancer* 2003;88:63–73.
18. Ferlay J, Bray F, Pisan P, Parkin DM. *Globocan 2000 and Globocan 2002: cancer incidence, mortality and prevalence worldwide*. Lyon: IARC Press, 2002.
19. World Health Organization. World Health Report Annex Table. 2004;3:128.
20. World Health Organization and International Agency for Research on Cancer. The current status of development of prophylactic vaccines against human papillomavirus infection. Technical Meeting Report, Geneva, 16–18 February 1999.
21. Mahdavi A, Monk BJ. Vaccines against human papillomavirus and cervical cancer: promises and challenges. *Oncologist* 2005;10:528–538.
22. Katz IT, Wright AA. Preventing cervical cancer in the developing world. *N Engl J Med* 2006;354:1110.
23. European Cervical Cancer Association. Cervical cancer in Europe. Fact Sheet 1V, March 2006.
24. Guzman CS, Salas RP, Puente PR, Hott AH, Israel AE, Guzman SR. Pesquisa y control del cáncer cérvico-uterino en el Servicio de Salud de Valdivia (1993–2003). *Rev Med Chile* 2005;133:685–692.
25. Denny L. The prevention of cervical cancer in developing countries. *BJOG* 2005;112:1204–1212.
26. Lewis MJ. A Situational Analysis of Cervical Cancer in Latin America and the Caribbean. Washington, DC: Pan American Health Organization, 2004.
27. American Social Health Association, National HPV and Cervical Cancer Prevention Center. HPV Background Information. Available at http://www.ashastd.org/learn/learn_hpv_bkgd.cfm.
28. Christensen ND, Reed CA, Cladel NM, Han R, et al. Immunization with virus-like particles induces long-term protection of rabbits against challenge with cottontail rabbit papillomavirus. *J Virol* 1996;70:960–965.
29. Harro CD, Pang YY, Roden RB, et al. Safety and immunogenicity trial in adult volunteers of a human papillomavirus 16 L1 virus-like particle. *J Natl Cancer Inst* 2001;93:284–292.
30. Koutsky LA, Ault KA, Wheeler CM, DR Brown CM, et al. A controlled trial of a human papillomavirus type 16 vaccine. *N Engl J Med* 2002;347(21):1645–1651.
31. Villa LL, Costa RLR, Petta CA, Andrade RP, et al. Prophylactic quadrivalent human papillomavirus [types 6, 11, 16 and 18] L1 virus-like particle vaccine in

young women: a randomized double-blind placebo-controlled multicentre phase 11 efficacy trial. *Lancet* 2005;6:271–278.

32. Merck's Investigational Vaccine GARDASIL Prevented 100 Percent of Cervical Pre-cancers and Non-invasive Cervical Cancers Associated with HPV Types 16 and 18 in New Clinical Study. Phase III Study Will Be Presented for the First Time at IDSA. Press release, October 6, 2005.

33. Muñoz N. For the FUTURE II Study Group. Efficacy of a quadrivalent HPV [types 6, 11, 16, 18] L1 VLP vaccine against cervical intraepithelial neoplasia grades 1-3 and adenocarcinoma in situ: a combined analysis. In: *Human papillomavirus infection and global prevention of cervical cancer.* EUROGIN 2006, Abstract SS 15-1.

34. Harper DM, Franco EL, Wheeler C, Ferris DG, et al. Efficacy of a bivalent L1-virus-like particle vaccine in prevention of infection with human papillomavirus types 16 and 18 in young women: a randomized controlled trial. *Lancet* 2004;364:1757–1765.

35. Harper DM, Franco EL, Wheeler CM, Mosciki AB, et al. Sustained efficacy up to 4.5 years of a bivalent L1 virus-like particle vaccine against human papillomavirus types 16 and 18: follow-up from a randomized control trial. *Lancet* 2006;367:1247–1255. Available at http://www.thelancet.com/Last accessed on April 15, 2006.

36. Goldie SJ, Gaffikin L, Goldhaber-Fiebert JD, Gordillo-Tobar A, et al. Cost effectiveness of cervical cancer screening in five developing countries. *N Engl J Med* 2005;353:2158–2168.

37. Goldie SJ, Kuhn L, Denny L, Pollack A, et al. Policy analysis of cervical cancer screening strategies in low-resource settings. *JAMA* 2001;285:3107–3115.

38. Brown ML, Goldie SJ, Draisma G, et al. Health service interventions for cancer control in developing countries. In: Jamison DT, Breman JG, Measham AR, Alleyne GAO, et al., eds. *Disease control priorities in developing countries,* 2nd ed. Washington, DC: World Bank; 2006. Available at http://www. dcp2.org.

39. Sanders GD, Taira AV. Cost-effectiveness of a potential vaccine for human papillomavirus. *Emerg Infect Dis.* January 2003;online serial.

40. Goldie SJ, Kohli M, Grima D, Weinstein MC, et al. Projected clinical benefits and cost-effectiveness of a human papillomavirus 16–18 vaccine. *J Natl Cancer Inst* 2004;96:604–615.

41. Kulasingam SL, Myers ER. Potential health and economic impact of adding human papillomavirus vaccine to screening programs. *JAMA* 2003;290:781–789.

42. World Health Organization. WHO consultation on human papillomavirus vaccines. *Wly Epidemiol Rec* 2005;80:297–304.

43. Kane M, Sherris J, Coursaget P, Aguado T, Cutts F. HPV vaccine use in the developing world. In: Bosch FX, et al., eds. *HPV vaccines and screening for cervical cancer prevention.* September 2006.